Dysrhythmia Recognition
and Man

D0760734

Karen Fenstermacher, MS, RN-C, FNP

Family Nurse Practitioner
Freeman Professional Center
Carthage, Missouri

SAUNDERS
An Imprint of Elsevier Science

The Curtis Center
Independence Square West
Philadelphia, Pennsylvania 19106

Library of Congress Cataloging-in-Publication Data

Fenstermacher, Karen.
    Dysrhythmia recognition and management / Karen Fenstermacher. — 3rd ed.
        p.   cm.
    Includes bibliographical references and index.
    ISBN 0–7216–7923–4
    1. Arrhythmia.   2. Electrocardiography.   I. Title.
    [DNLM: 1. Arrhythmia—diagnosis handbooks.   2. Arrhythmia—drug
therapy handbooks.   3. Electrocardiography handbooks.   WG 39 F341d 1998]
RC685.A65F36   1998
616.1'28—dc21
DNLM/DLC   98–5491

DYSRHYTHMIA RECOGNITION AND MANAGEMENT, 3rd edition   ISBN 0–7216–7923–4

Printed in the United States of America

Last digit is the print number: 9   8   7   6   5   4   3

NOTICE

In preparing this text, the author has made every effort to verify the drug selections and standard dosages presented herein. It is not intended as a source of specific or correct drug use or dosage for any patient. Because of changes in government regulations, research findings, and other information related to drug therapy and drug reactions, it is essential for the reader to check the information and instructions provided by the manufacturer for each drug and therapeutic agent. These may reflect changes in indications or dosage and/or contain relevant warnings and precautions. Attention to these details is particularly important when the recommended agent is a new and/or infrequently employed drug. Any discrepancies or errors should be brought to the attention of the publisher.

◣ Preface

This book is a concise yet complete guide to most of the dysrhythmias that are seen by nurses, physicians, monitor technicians, paramedics, and students practicing in critical care or emergency departments, telemetry stepdown or postanesthesia units, and outpatient clinics. The electrocardiogram (ECG) changes that are the criteria for recognizing dysrhythmias are highlighted throughout. Sample ECG strips are given in leads II and MCL_1 for most rhythms to provide both the student and experienced practitioner with a more complete understanding of the rhythm. Dysrhythmias are also considered in terms of causes and treatments. Hence, sections are included on basic cardiac physiology, advanced cardiac life support (ACLS) algorithms, and emergency cardiovascular drugs. Drug dosages and treatments follow the current 1992 ACLS protocols.

The 12-lead ECG section includes normal 12-lead interpretation as well as bundle branch block, myocardial infarction (including right ventricular infarction), and chamber hypertrophy. This section has been expanded to include advanced rhythm analysis for digitalis toxicity and for differentiating ectopy and aberrancy. A glossary of terms provides further detail. Although most 12-lead ECGs are computer generated and "interpreted," the staff, especially in critical care areas, must know whether the interpretation is correct (which oftentimes it is not).

Dysrhythmia Recognition and Management is intended as a memory aid and review for both students and experienced practitioners. Textbooks, which are more comprehensive, introduce this subject and provide practice strips necessary to sharpen one's interpretive skills as well. Textbooks, however, also include much additional information not necessary for rhythm interpretation. In addition, they are more expensive and not as portable.

◤ Acknowledgments

I want to dedicate this edition to my parents, Dale and Ann, and to thank my family, friends, and coworkers for their continued support in my professional endeavors.

Karen Fenstermacher

ABOUT THE AUTHOR

Ms. Fenstermacher has been a nurse for 20 years, practicing primarily in critical care areas (intensive care, cardiovascular intensive care, and emergency department). She also has 5 years experience in education and has much experience teaching basic and advanced ECG interpretation and ACLS courses. She is currently a family nurse practitioner working in a private clinic.

◤ Contents

Conduction System / 2
Intervals and Waveforms / 4
Intervals and Rates / 6
Natural Pacemakers / 10
Monitoring Leads / 12
Lead Wires Reversed / 14
Factors Contributing to Dysrhythmias / 16
Rhythm Strip Interpretation / 18
Normal Sinus Rhythm (NSR) / 20
Sinus Bradycardia / 24
Sinus Tachycardia / 26
Sinus Dysrhythmia / 28
Sinus Exit Block (Second-Degree SA Block, Type II) / 30
Sinus Arrest / 32
Sick Sinus Syndrome (Bradycardia-Tachycardia Syndrome) / 34
Premature Atrial Contraction (PAC) / 36
Wandering Atrial Pacemaker / 38

Multifocal Atrial Tachycardia (MAT) / 40
Atrial Flutter / 42
Atrial Fibrillation / 44
Premature Junctional Contraction (PJC) / 48
Junctional Rhythm / 50
Accelerated Junctional Rhythm / 54
Supraventricular Tachycardia (SVT) / 58
Premature Ventricular Contraction (PVC) / 60
Ventricular Tachycardia (V-Tach) / 64
Torsades de Pointes / 68
Ventricular Fibrillation (V-Fib) / 70
Asystole / 72
Idioventricular Rhythm / 74
Accelerated Idioventricular Rhythm / 76
First-Degree AV Block / 78
Second-Degree AV Block, Mobitz I (Wenckebach) / 80
Second-Degree AV Block, Mobitz II / 84

Third-Degree (Complete) AV Block / 88
Differentiating AV Blocks / 92
AV Dissociation / 93
Emergency Cardiac Drugs / 94
  Mechanism of Action: Catecholamines / 95
  Mechanism of Action: Antiarrhythmic
      Medications / 96
  Adenosine (Adenocard) / 98
  Amrinone (Inocor) / 99
  Atropine / 100
  Bretylium (Bretylol) / 101
  Calcium Chloride / 102
  Digoxin (Lanoxin) / 103
  Diltiazem (Cardizem) / 104
  dl–Sotalol (Betapace) / 105
  Dobutamine (Dobutrex) / 106
  Dopamine (Intropin) / 107
  Epinephrine (Adrenalin) / 108
  Ibutilide Fumarate (Corvert) / 110

Isoproterenol (Isuprel) / 111
Lidocaine / 112
Magnesium Sulfate / 113
Morphine / 114
Procainamide (Pronestyl, Procan SR) / 115
Propranolol (Inderal) / 116
Quinidine / 117
Sodium Bicarbonate / 118
Verapamil (Calan, Isoptin) / 119
ACLS Algorithms / 120
  Ventricular Fibrillation—Pulseless
      Ventricular Tachycardia / 122
  Ventricular Tachycardia/Wide-QRS
      Tachycardia / 124
  Electrical Cardioversion (for Patient with
      Pulse) / 126
  Pulseless Electrical Activity (PEA) / 128
  Asystole / 130

Bradycardia / **132**
Supraventricular Tachycardia / **134**
12-Lead ECG / **136**
Limb Leads / **137**
Precordial Leads / **138**
Axis Determination / **140**
Normal 12-Lead ECG / **142**
Atrial Abnormalities / **144**
Right Atrial Abnormality (P pulmonale) / **144**
Left Atrial Abnormality (P mitrale) / **146**
Ventricular Hypertrophy / **148**
Right Ventricular Hypertrophy (RVH) / **150**
Left Ventricular Hypertrophy (LVH) / **152**
Myocardial Infarction / **154**
Q Wave Infarction / **154**
ECG Changes / **156**
Anterior Myocardial Infarction / **158**

Septal Myocardial Infarction / **160**
Inferior Myocardial Infarction / **162**
Right Ventricular Infarction / **165**
Lateral Myocardial Infarction / **168**
Posterior Myocardial Infarction / **170**
Non-Q-Wave Myocardial Infarction / **172**
Critical LAD Stenosis (Wellens Syndrome) / **174**
Bundle Branch Block (BBB) / **178**
Differentiating Ectopy and Aberrancy / **182**
QRS Configurations in Wide-QRS Tachycardia / **184**
Digitalis Toxicity / **186**
Junctional Tachycardia (Nonparoxysmal) / **189**
Atrial Tachycardia with Block / **190**
Glossary / **192**
References / **204**
Index / **210**

Dysrhythmia Recognition *and* Management

Conduction System

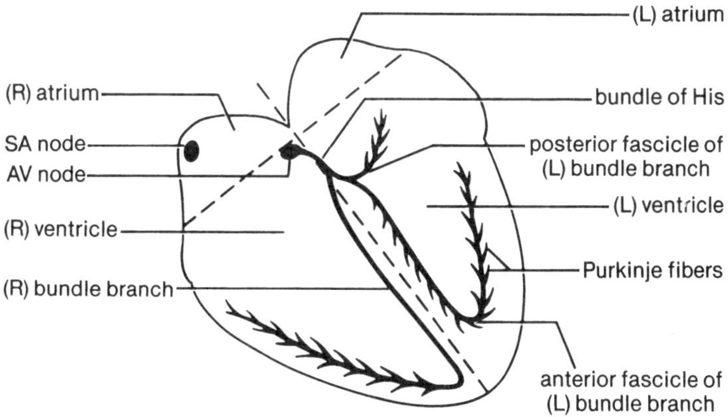
(L) atrium
(R) atrium
bundle of His
SA node
AV node
posterior fascicle of
(L) bundle branch
(L) ventricle
(R) ventricle
Purkinje fibers
(R) bundle branch
anterior fascicle of
(L) bundle branch

NORMAL CONDUCTION

The electrical impulse normally originates in the sinoatrial (SA) node and spreads throughout the atrial muscle to the atrioventricular (AV) node. The atria then contract. The impulse slows slightly in the AV node and then continues through the bundle of His and the right and left bundle branches to the Purkinje fibers and through the ventricular muscle. The ventricles then contract. The spread of the electrical impulse before contraction is known as depolarization; there is atrial depolarization and ventricular depolarization. Depolarization is followed by repolarization, which is the "resting state" of myocardial cells. Here they prepare themselves for another depolarization. One depolarization followed by a full repolarization is known as one cardiac cycle.

The electrical impulses from the heart are depicted as positive (upright) waveforms or negative (downward) waveforms on electrocardiogram (ECG) recording paper.

◣ Intervals and Waveforms

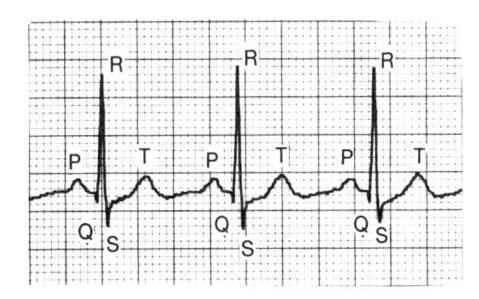

P Wave impulse spreading through atria (atrial depolarization*)
QRS impulse spreading through ventricles (ventricular depolarization*)
    Q wave is the negative deflection before the R wave
    R wave is first positive deflection after the P wave
    S wave is the negative deflection after the R wave
T Wave ventricular repolarization* (there is atrial repolarization, but usually it is obscured by the
        QRS complex)

---

*Refer to glossary for more information.

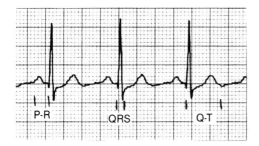

PR Interval time it takes for the impulse to spread from the SA node through the atrial muscle and the AV node; it is measured from the beginning of the P wave to the beginning of the QRS

QRS Interval time it takes for the impulse to spread through the right and left ventricles; it is measured from the beginning of the QRS to the end of the QRS

QT Interval time it takes for the impulse to spread through the ventricles and for repolarization to occur; it is measured from the beginning of the QRS to the end of the T wave

5

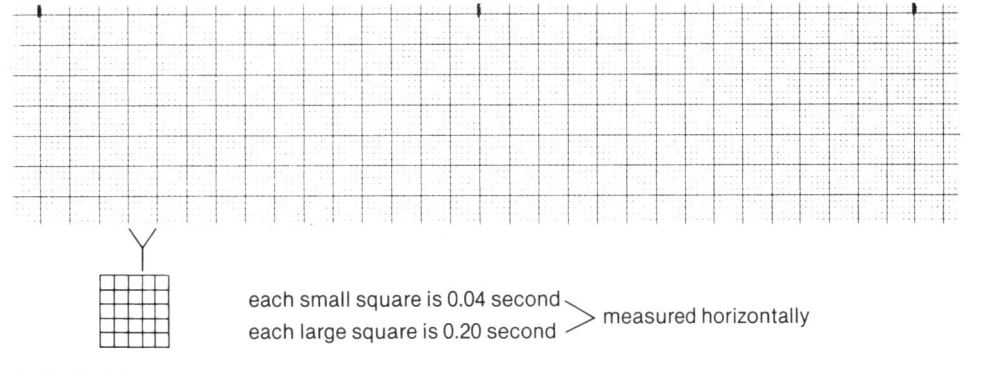

each small square is 0.04 second
each large square is 0.20 second
} measured horizontally

INTERVALS

A PR interval of three small squares (horizontally) is 0.12 second. Measured vertically, each small square is 1 mm, which is used to determine ST depression or elevation as well as chamber strain or hypertrophy.*

*Refer to glossary for more information.

Normal Values

PR 0.12 to 0.20 s

QRS 0.04 to 0.10 s

QT 0.32 to 0.44 s

KEY POINTS • The QT interval can be affected by the heart rate (which may shorten as the rate increases), electrolyte imbalances, and some antiarrhythmics, especially quinidine, procainamide, and disopyramide (Norpace).

• The physician should be notified if the QT intervals begin lengthening.

Continued on following page

RATES

To calculate rates:
1. Count the number of R waves in a 6-second strip and multiply by 10. (The slashes at the top or bottom of the strips are at 3-second intervals.) This is the only choice if the rhythm is irregular.
2. For regular rhythms (requires memorization but is accurate):
   a. Find an R wave on a heavy line and call this line 0.
   b. Starting with the next heavy line, name each line you come across until the next R wave as follows: 300, 150, 100, 75, 60, 50.
   c. If the next R wave falls between heavy lines, determine the value for each little box between the two heavy lines and then calculate the rate (see example below).

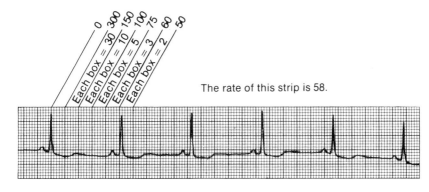

Each box = 0 — 30 — 300 — 10 — 150 — 5 — 100 — 3 — 75 — 2 — 60 — 50

The rate of this strip is 58.

KEY POINT The ventricular rate is calculated using R waves. The atrial rate can be calculated in the same manner using P waves.

9

◣ Natural Pacemakers

The SA node is known as the pacemaker of the heart. In a majority of people the SA node initiates most, if not all, of the electrical impulses. In the event that the SA node does not fire, the area of the conduction system with the highest rate assumes the role of pacing the heart.

Inherent or "Normal" Rates

SA Node 60 to 100 beats per minute (bpm)
AV Node 40 to 60 bpm
Ventricle 20 to 40 bpm

If the sinus node fails and no other part of the heart begins initiating impulses, the AV node will try, but only at the inherent rate of the AV node, which is 40 to 60 bpm. If the AV node also fails to fire, the ventricles will try to pace the heart at 20 to 40 bpm.

The illustrations show electrode placement and normal rhythm strip for leads II and MCL₁.

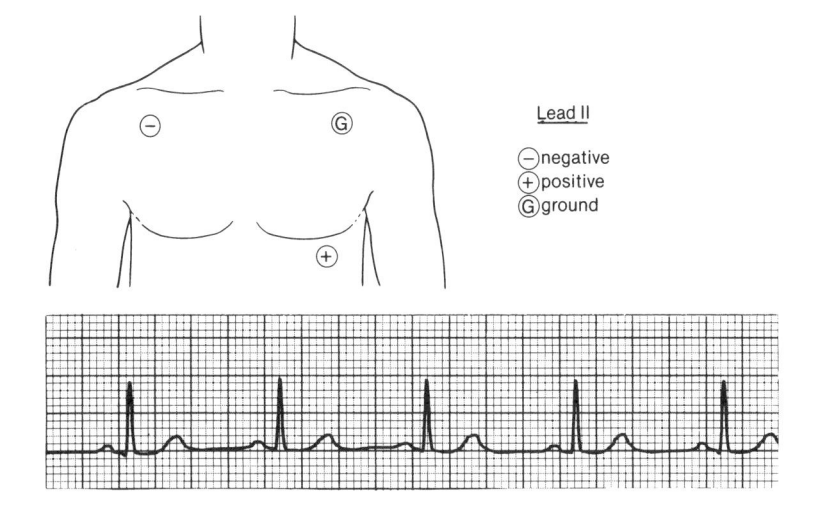

Lead II

⊖ negative
⊕ positive
Ⓖ ground

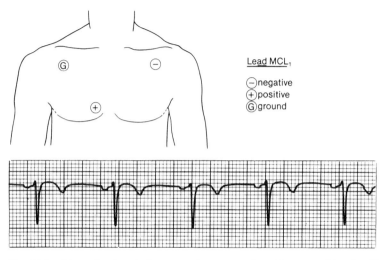

Lead MCL₁

⊖ negative
⊕ positive
Ⓖ ground

The ⊕ lead is at the fourth intercostal space on the right sternal border. For quick MCL_1 placement, set the lead selector for lead III and move the left leg electrode to the ⊕ position.

Lead II P wave upright
QRS mostly upright (positive)

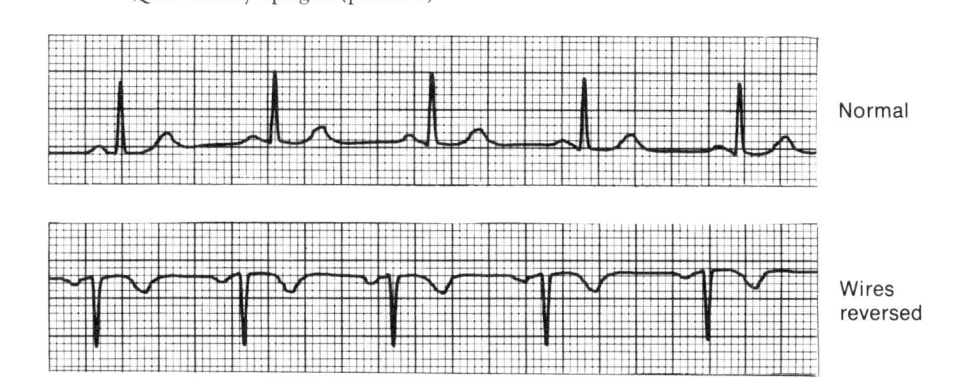

Normal

Wires
reversed

Lead MCL₁ P wave inverted or biphasic
QRS mostly negative

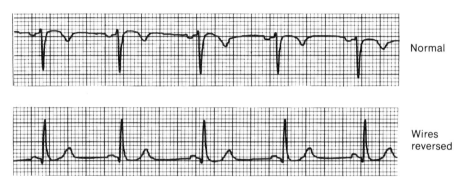

Normal

Wires
reversed

KEY POINT The ECG strip will appear "upside-down" when the positive and negative wires are reversed. The lead placement should be checked.

◼ Factors Contributing to Dysrhythmias

Potential Causes	Tachycardia	Ectopy*	Bradycardia	Conduction Delays
Myocardial infarction (MI), hypoxia	✓	✓	✓	✓
Mechanical stretch of tissue	✓	✓	✓	✓
Congestive heart failure (CHF)				
Chamber dilation or hypertrophy				
Excess catecholamines	✓	✓		
Stress				
Pain				
CHF				
Medications (e.g., dopamine, epinephrine)				
Severe metabolic alkalosis	✓	✓		
Vagal stimulation			✓	
Hyperkalemia			✓	✓
Hypokalemia	✓ (ventricular)	✓		✓

*Refer to glossary for more information.

To learn how to interpret ECG rhythms accurately, it is important to establish a pattern of consistent evaluation for each strip. A commonly used format follows:

P Waves Are they similar?
        Is there one, and only one, to each QRS?*
Rhythm Is the atrial rhythm (i.e., P wave to P wave) regular?
        Is the ventricular rhythm (i.e., R wave to R wave) regular?
        If the rhythm is irregular, is there a pattern?
Rate Atrial and ventricular
PR Interval duration in seconds[†]
QRS Interval duration in seconds[†]
QT Interval duration in seconds[†]

KEY POINT If there is only one P wave for each QRS, only one rhythm and rate need be measured; thus looking at P waves first can be a shortcut.

---

*When there is more than one atrial complex for each ventricular complex (as in atrial flutter or second-degree AV block), the conduction is stated as a ratio. For example, second-degree AV block with every other P wave conducted is evaluated as second-degree AV block with 2:1 conduction.
[†]Refer to page 7 for normal values.

◤ Normal Sinus Rhythm (NSR)

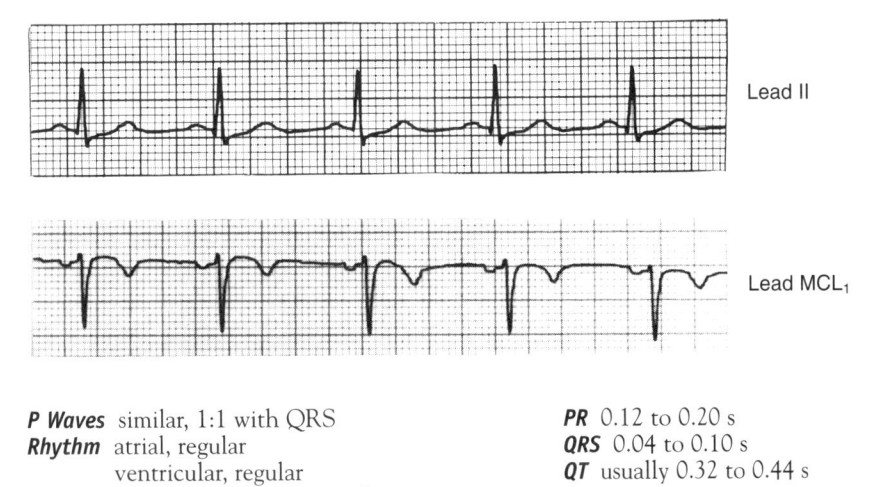

Lead II

Lead MCL$_1$

P Waves similar, 1:1 with QRS

Rhythm atrial, regular
ventricular, regular

Rate atrial, 60 to 100 bpm } same rate
ventricular, 60 to 100 bpm

PR 0.12 to 0.20 s

QRS 0.04 to 0.10 s

QT usually 0.32 to 0.44 s

Treatment none required

KEY POINT If the QRS or QT interval or both are abnormal but the other criteria for sinus rhythm are met, the evaluation would still be sinus rhythm (but with wide QRS or short QT, for example).

EXAMPLES OF SINUS RHYTHMS

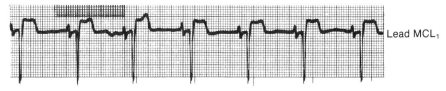

Lead MCL₁

Sinus rhythm.

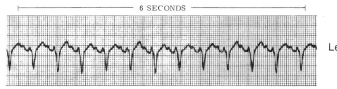

Lead II

Sinus tachycardia.

Continued on following page

21

■ Normal Sinus Rhythm (NSR) *(Continued)*

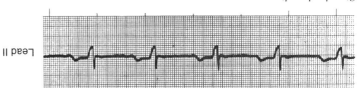

Lead MCL₁

|← 6 SECONDS →|

Sinus rhythm.

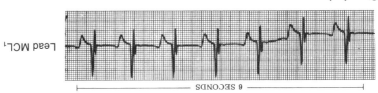

Lead II

Sinus bradycardia.

◣ Sinus Bradycardia

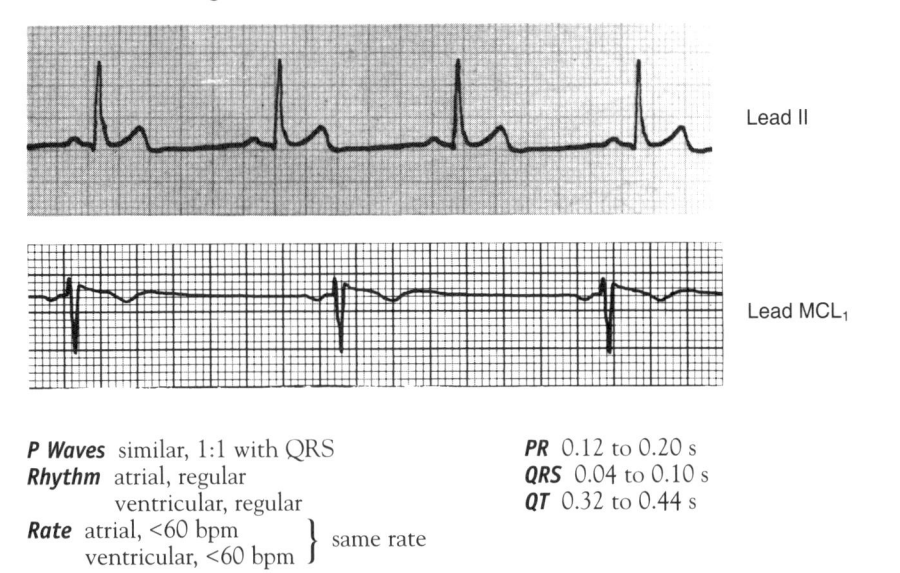

Lead II

Lead MCL₁

P Waves similar, 1:1 with QRS
Rhythm atrial, regular
ventricular, regular
Rate atrial, <60 bpm
ventricular, <60 bpm } same rate

PR 0.12 to 0.20 s
QRS 0.04 to 0.10 s
QT 0.32 to 0.44 s

Possible Causes vagal response (e.g., gagging, vomiting, straining)
drug effect (e.g., digoxin or beta blockers, such as propranolol)
good cardiovascular tone, as in an athlete
compensatory response in acute MI (especially inferior)
chronic ischemic heart disease
degenerative disease of the SA node (sick sinus syndrome)
hypothyroidism
increased intracranial pressure

Treatment 1. instituted if patient is symptomatic:
   - systolic blood pressure (BP) <90 mm Hg
   - heart rate <60 bpm
   - skin cool and clammy
   - premature ventricular contractions (PVCs)
   - chest pain
   - dyspnea
   2. atropine 0.5 to 1 mg IV push; can be repeated every 3 to 5 minutes up to 3 mg total*
   (See Bradycardia Algorithm [p. 132] for continued therapy.)

---

*For more information on drug therapy, refer to drug section.

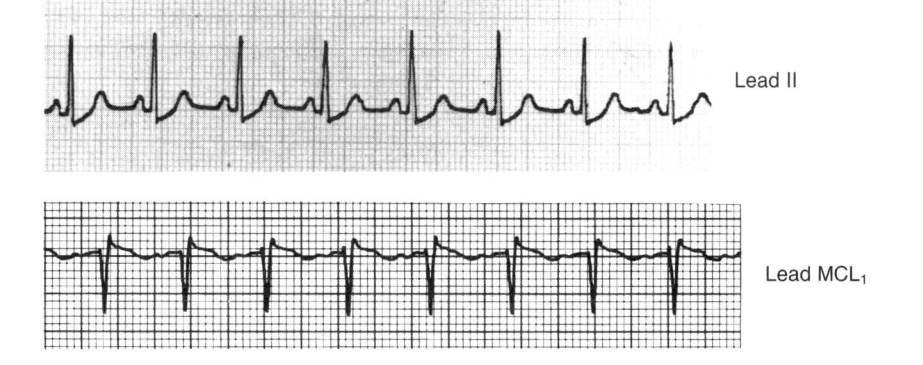

Lead II

Lead MCL₁

P Waves similar, 1:1 with QRS
Rhythm atrial, regular
       ventricular, regular
Rate atrial, 100 to 150 bpm ⎫
      ventricular, 100 to 150 bpm ⎭ same rate

PR 0.12 to 0.20 s
QRS 0.04 to 0.10 s
QT 0.32 to 0.44 s

Possible Causes	anxiety	exercise	hypovolemia
	pain	caffeine	hypotension
	hypoxia	nicotine	acute MI
	fear	alcohol	amphetamines
	fright	fever	thyroid supplements
	anger	anemia	heart disease, e.g., CHF
	hyperthyroidism		

Treatment
1. treat underlying cause
2. verapamil, digitalis, or beta-blocker may be used if rhythm is causing hemodynamic instability*

KEY POINT Sinus tachycardia is normal in infants and young children but is not found in adults without a cause.

---

*For more information on drug therapy, refer to drug section.

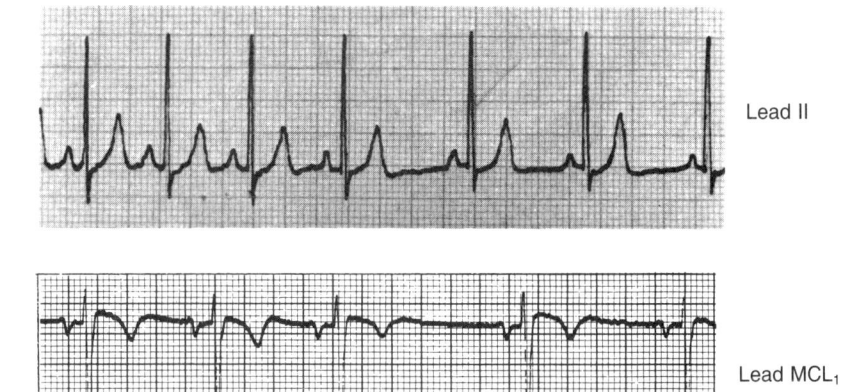

Lead II

Lead MCL₁

P Waves usually similar, 1:1 with QRS

Rhythm atrial, irregular ⎫ often associated with breathing;
ventricular, irregular ⎭ slows on inspiration

Rate atrial, 60 to 100 bpm ⎫ same rate
ventricular, 60 to 100 bpm ⎭

PR 0.12 to 0.20 s

QRS 0.04 to 0.10 s

QT 0.32 to 0.44 s

Possible Causes respirations
sick sinus syndrome
alteration in vagal tone (e.g., stooping, bearing down, or vomiting)

Treatment none; fairly common in children

◼ Sinus Exit Block (Second-Degree SA Block, Type II)

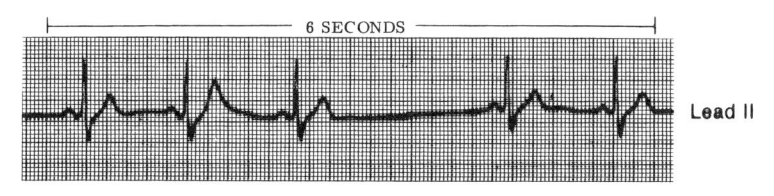

Lead II

P Waves similar, 1:1 with QRS
Rhythm atrial, regular except for pause
        ventricular, regular except for pause
Rate usually 60 to 100 bpm (basic rhythm)
PR 0.12 to 0.20 s
QRS 0.04 to 0.10 s
QT 0.32 to 0.44 s

Possible Causes   excessive vagal stimulation
acute MI or myocarditis
scar tissue
drug therapy (e.g., beta blockers, digitalis, calcium channel blockers, and amiodarone)

Treatment   usually none is needed; if symptomatic, atropine 0.5 mg IV may be given*

KEY POINT The hallmark of sinus exit block is a pause that is a multiple of the normal PP interval, usually twice as long, but it can be longer.

---

*For more information on drug therapy, refer to drug section.

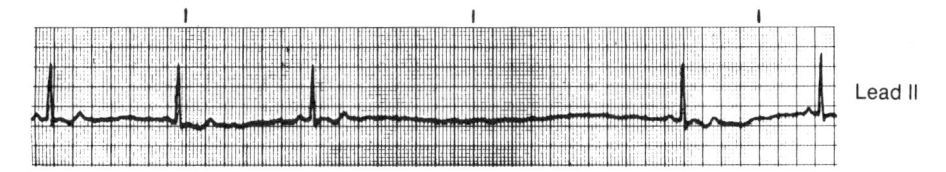

Lead II

P Waves similar, 1:1 with QRS
Rhythm atrial, irregular because of pause
       ventricular, irregular because of pause
Rate depends on number and lengths of pauses
PR 0.12 to 0.20 s
QRS 0.04 to 0.10 s
QT 0.32 to 0.44 s

Possible Causes   excessive vagal stimulation
acute MI
fibrosis of conduction system
hyperkalemia or hypokalemia
digitalis intoxication (see p. 186)
drug therapy (e.g., class IA or IC antiarrhythmics and amiodarone)

Treatment   1. if ventricular rate is too slow or pauses are frequent, atropine may be given to stimulate SA node*
2. temporary or permanent pacemaker is often indicated

KEY POINT The hallmark of sinus arrest is a pause that is not a multiple of the normal PP interval.

---

*For more information on drug therapy, refer to drug section.

◣ Sick Sinus Syndrome (Bradycardia-Tachycardia Syndrome)

ECG Changes alternating periods of bradycardia with tachycardia; each rhythm may be sustained for an indeterminate time

Causes disease within the SA node
conduction failure between SA node and atrial tissue

Possible Symptoms may be varied or intermittent or both; syncope, dizziness, palpitations, more frequent or intense angina, worsened CHF, cerebral embolism

Treatment 1. permanent pacemaker (especially with persistent, symptomatic bradycardia)
2. digoxin may be used for atrial tachydysrhythmias*

Precautions treatment of atrial fibrillation (A-fib) in sick sinus syndrome can cause severe bradycardia

---

*Refer to glossary for more information.

◥ Premature Atrial Contraction (PAC)

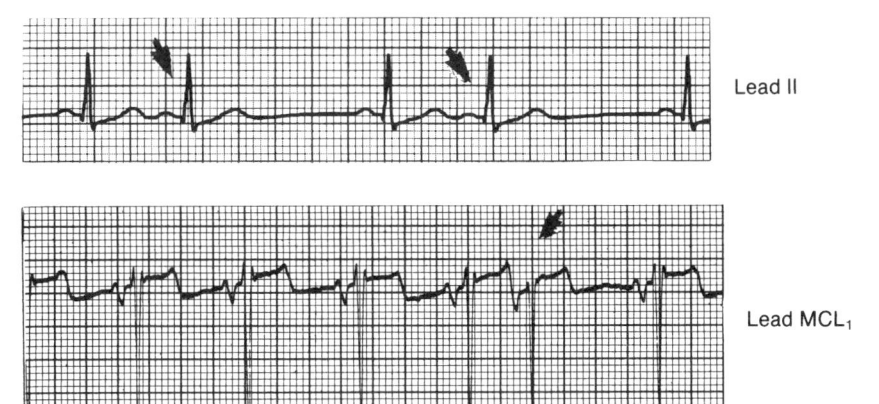

Lead II

Lead MCL₁

P Waves P wave of PAC is different, 1:1 with QRS

Rhythm atrial, irregular ⎱ because of premature beat;
ventricular, irregular ⎰ basic rhythm is regular

Rate atrial ⎱ of basic rhythm usually 60 to 100 bpm
ventricular ⎰

PR may be normal (0.12 to 0.20 s) or prolonged

QRS normally 0.04 to 0.10 s; wide with aberrant ventricular conduction*

QT 0.32 to 0.44 s

Possible Causes stimulants (caffeine, tobacco, alcohol)
hypoxia
digitalis intoxication (see p. 186)
CHF
anxiety
atrial enlargement

Treatment 1. usually none, but be aware that PACs can initiate other tachydysrhythmias* (e.g., A-fib)
2. withhold caffeine, tobacco, and so on

---

*Refer to glossary for more information

■ Wandering Atrial Pacemaker

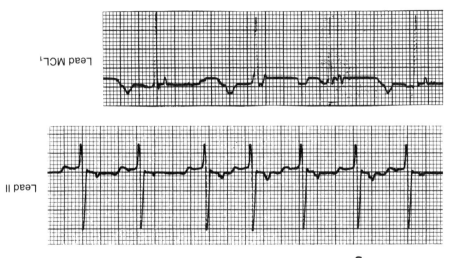

Lead MCL₁

Lead II

P Waves dissimilar, have different configurations; 1:1 with QRS, but PP intervals often vary

Rhythm atrial, regular or slightly irregular
    ventricular, regular or slightly irregular

Rate atrial, usually 60 to 100 bpm } same rate
    ventricular, usually 60 to 100 bpm }

PR 0.12 to 0.20 s; may vary with different P waves

QRS 0.04 to 0.10 s

QT 0.32 to 0.44 s

Treatment none usually needed

Multifocal Atrial Tachycardia (MAT)

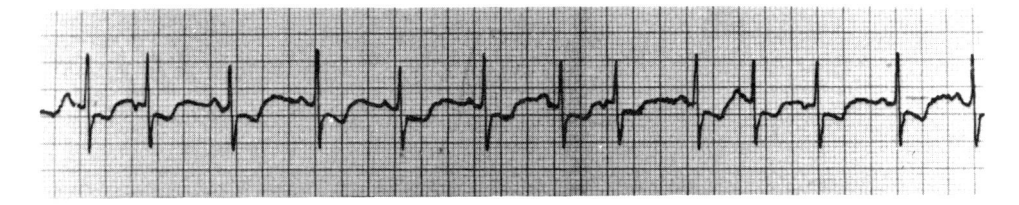

Lead II

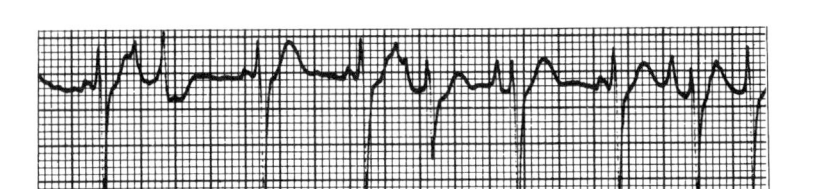

Lead MCL₁

P Waves change configuration with almost every beat; 1:1 with QRS

Rhythm atrial, irregular
ventricular, irregular

Rate atrial, >100 bpm
ventricular, >100 bpm $\Big\}$ same rate

PR 0.12 to 0.20 s but changes beat to beat

QRS 0.04 to 0.10 s; complexes can vary in configuration

QT 0.32 to 0.44 s

Possible Causes serious illness, usually associated with chronic lung disease or metabolic disturbances, e.g., hypoxemia or hypokalemia

Treatment 1. directed at primary cause, e.g., chronic obstructive pulmonary disease (COPD), CHF, or electrolyte imbalance
2. MAT is resistant to digitalis therapy

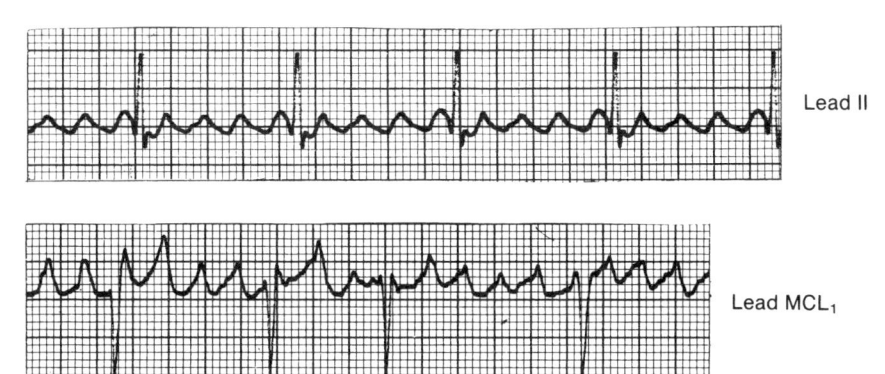

Lead II

Lead MCL₁

P Waves none; "F" or flutter waves (sawtooth)
Rhythm atrial, regular
       ventricular, usually regular with constant conduction ratio*; irregular otherwise
Rate atrial, usually 280 to 320 bpm
    ventricular, depends on conduction through to ventricles

PR none
QRS 0.04 to 0.10 s
QT 0.32 to 0.44 s

Possible Causes rarely occurs in the absence of organic heart disease (e.g., rheumatic or valvular disease, chronic ischemic or hypertensive disease, atrial hypertrophy*); may occur in toxic or metabolic conditions that affect the heart (e.g., thyrotoxicosis, alcoholism, beriberi)

Treatment 1. digitalis to decrease AV conduction and slow the ventricular rate[†]
2. cardioversion* or atrial pacing
3. verapamil not recommended because it has caused 1:1 conduction in atrial flutter
(See Supraventricular Tachycardia Algorithm [p. 134] for continued therapy.)

KEY POINTS The most common conduction ratio is 2:1, and the second most common ratio is 4:1.

---

*Refer to glossary for more information.
[†]For more information on drug therapy, refer to drug section.

Lead MCL₁

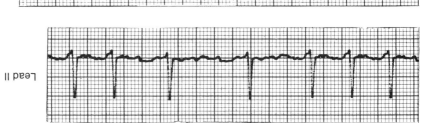

Lead II

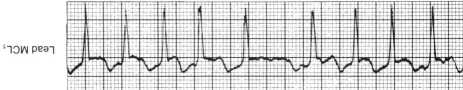

P Waves none; "f" or fibrillatory waves (atria "quiver," no organized contraction)
Rhythm atrial, totally irregular
         ventricular, totally irregular
Rate atrial, >400 bpm (uncountable)
     ventricular, <100 bpm (controlled A-fib)
                   >100 bpm (uncontrolled A-fib)

PR none
QRS 0.04 to 0.10 s
QT 0.32 to 0.44 s

Possible Causes usually the result of underlying heart disease (e.g., rheumatic or valvular disease, chronic ischemic or hypertensive disease, atrial hypertrophy,* and pericarditis); other possible causes are

digitalis intoxication (see p. 186)
hypoxia
alcohol excess
cigarette smoking
common in COPD
acute MI

---

*Refer to glossary for more information.

Continued on following page

Treatment **1.** depends on the ventricular rate (the goal of therapy is to convert to normal sinus rhythm [NSR] or at least to decrease the ventricular rate to <100 bpm) and on how patient tolerates the loss of "atrial kick"*

2. radiofrequency (RF) ablation* of the His bundle may be used with drug-resistant cases; this will slow the ventricular rate but does not remove the chance of thromboembolism

3. often ibutilide fumarate or diltiazem is administered intravenously for conversion of acute onset A-fib†

KEY POINTS
- Despite the ventricular rate, the physician should be notified when the patient goes into A-fib so that conversion to NSR can be achieved as soon as possible.
- A-fib may occur intermittently or as a chronic rhythm.
- A-fib is often preceded by PACs or atrial tachycardia; after conversion, the patient may continue to have atrial ectopic* rhythms.

---

*Refer to glossary for more information.
†For information on drug therapy, refer to drug section.

Premature Junctional Contraction (PJC)

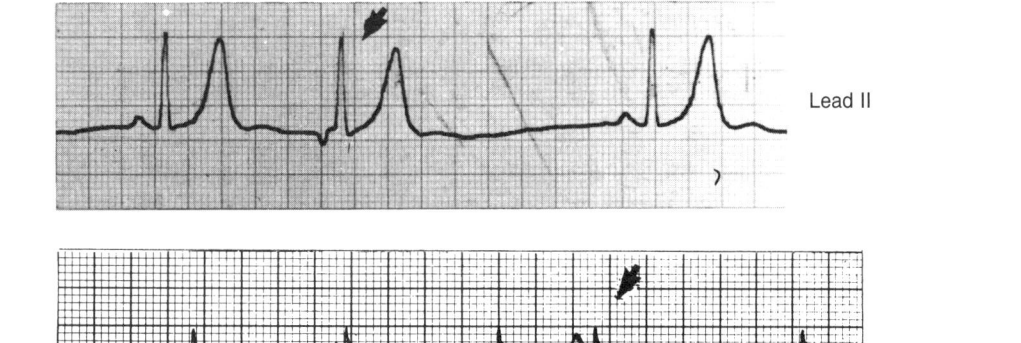

Lead II

Lead MCL₁

P Waves similar except for PJC, which may be absent or different (see Key Points below); 1:1 with QRS

Rhythm atrial, irregular ⎫ because of premature beat;
ventricular, irregular ⎭ basic rhythm is regular

Rate usually 40 to 100 bpm (basic rhythm)

PR 0.12 to 0.20 s; when present, PR of PJC is usually shortened

QRS 0.04 to 0.10 s

QT 0.32 to 0.44 s

Possible Causes digitalis intoxication (see p. 186) CHF ischemia or acute MI tobacco
alcohol hypoxia caffeine

Treatment none usually needed

KEY POINTS: In a junctional rhythm the impulse originates in or near the AV node and is conducted retrogradely to the atria as well as down to the ventricles.
- If the impulse spreads through the atria first, the P wave will be inverted before the QRS in lead II; in lead MCL$_1$ the PR will be short (<0.12 s).
- If the impulse spreads through the atria and ventricles simultaneously, the P wave will be buried within the QRS, so it will not be visible.
- If the impulse spreads through the ventricles first, the P wave will be inverted after the QRS in lead II; in lead MCL$_1$ the P wave is usually upright but occurs after the QRS.

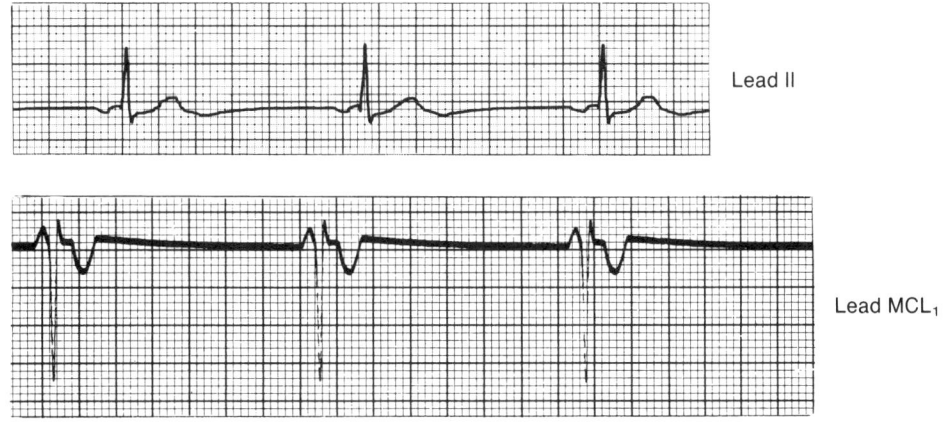

P Waves *lead II:* none, or inverted before or after QRS
lead MCL₁: none, or usually upright but with PR <0.12 s

Rhythm atrial, regular when present
ventricular, regular

Rate atrial, 40 to 60 bpm
ventricular, 40 to 60 bpm $\Big\}$ same rate

PR usually <0.12 s when present

QRS 0.04 to 0.10 s

QT 0.32 to 0.44 s

Possible Causes increased vagal tone   acute MI
beta blocker (e.g., propranolol)   as an escape rhythm in second- or
rheumatic heart disease   third-degree AV block
digitalis intoxication (see p. 186)

Treatment none unless the rate is too slow for the patient to tolerate or the loss of "atrial kick"*
causes instability; then atropine 0.5 mg IV push may be given†

---

*Refer to glossary for more information.
†For more information on drug therapy, refer to drug section.

Continued on following page

KEY POINTS In a junctional rhythm the impulse originates in or near the AV node and is conducted retrogradely to the atria as well as down to the ventricles.

- If the impulse spreads through the atria first, the P wave will be inverted before the QRS in lead II; in lead MCL_1 the PR will be short (<0.12 s).
- If the impulse spreads through the atria and ventricles simultaneously, the P wave will be buried within the QRS, so it will not be visible.
- If the impulse spreads through the ventricles first, the P wave will be inverted after the QRS in lead II; in lead MCL_1 the P wave is usually upright but occurs after the QRS.

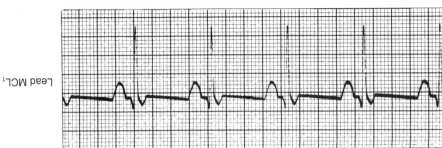

Lead MCL₁

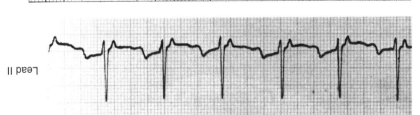

Lead II

P Waves *lead II*: none, or inverted before or after QRS
lead MCL_1: none, or usually upright but with a PR <0.12 s

Rhythm atrial, regular when present
ventricular, regular

Rate 60 to 100 bpm

PR usually <0.12 s when present

QRS 0.04 to 0.10 s

QT 0.32 to 0.44 s

Possible Causes occurs with high frequency in acute MI (especially inferior wall) digitalis intoxication (see p. 186) increased vagal tone as an escape rhythm in second- and third-degree AV block

Treatment 1. none unless the patient does not tolerate the loss of "atrial kick"*; then atropine 0.5 mg IV push†
2. if caused by digoxin, aggressively manage the toxicity (see p. 186)

---

*Refer to glossary for more information.
†For more information on drug therapy, refer to drug section.

Continued on following page

KEY POINTS In a junctional rhythm the impulse originates in or near the AV node and is conducted retrogradely to the atria as well as down to the ventricles.

- If the impulse spreads through the atria first, the P wave will be inverted before the QRS in lead II; in lead MCL_1 the PR will be short (<0.12 s).
- If the impulse spreads through the atria and ventricles simultaneously, the P wave will be buried within the QRS, so it will not be visible.
- If the impulse spreads through the ventricles first, the P wave will be inverted after the QRS in lead II; in lead MCL_1 the P wave is usually upright but occurs after the QRS.

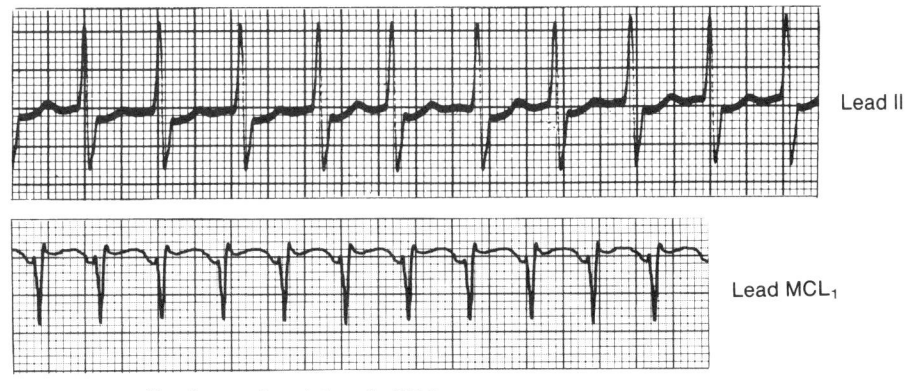

Lead II

Lead MCL₁

P Waves usually obscure but 1:1 with QRS
Rhythm regular
Rate 150 to 250 bpm
PR 0.12 to 0.20 s when present
QRS 0.04 to 0.10 s; can be aberrantly conducted* through ventricles
QT usually 0.32 to 0.44 s

Possible Causes digitalis intoxication (see p. 186)   rheumatic heart disease
                      chronic ischemic heart disease   acute MI
                      mitral valve prolapse   hypoxia
                      hyperthyroidism   reentry* within AV node
                      associated with preexcitation syndromes* (e.g., Wolff-Parkinson-White or
                         Lown-Ganong-Levine syndromes)
                      sympathomimetic agents (i.e., dopamine, epinephrine, isoproterenol)†

Treatment depends on ventricular rate and on patient's being hemodynamically stable (i.e.,
                 stable vital signs, dry skin, no dizziness or syncope)
                 (See Supraventricular Tachycardia Algorithm [p. 134] for continued therapy.)

KEY POINTS The term "supraventricular tachycardia" is a catchall for a rhythm with questionable
atrial activity but with a normal QRS width (indicating it originates above the ventricles). The
term should be used only when a more definitive diagnosis (e.g., atrial tachycardia or A-fib)
cannot be made. When this rhythm suddenly starts or stops, it is called paroxysmal SVT or
PSVT (formerly called PAT).

---

*Refer to glossary for more information.
†For information on drug therapy, refer to drug section.

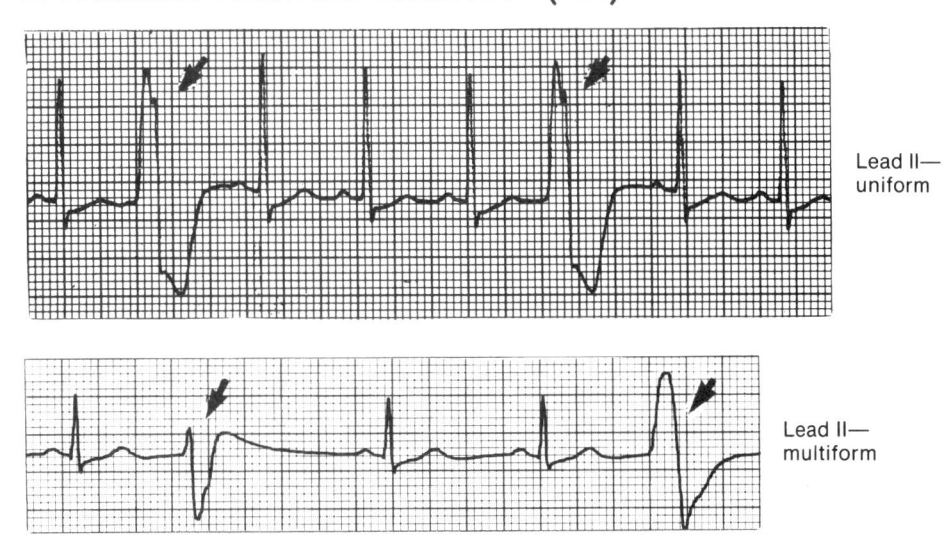

Lead II—
uniform

Lead II—
multiform

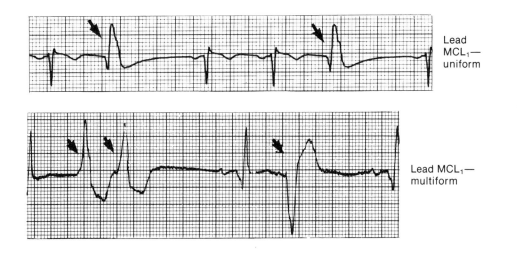

Lead MCL$_1$—uniform

Lead MCL$_1$—multiform

Continued on following page

If the PVCs originate from one focus, they are uniform.*
If the PVCs originate from more than one focus, they are multiform.*

P Waves usually none seen before premature ventricular complex, but normal with basic rhythm

Rhythm atrial, irregular⎫ because of premature beat or beats;
ventricular, irregular⎭ basic rhythm is regular

QRS, ST, T Wave QRS > 0.12 s and bizarre configuration
ST and T wave opposite of QRS
full compensatory pause* is usual

Possible Causes reentry phenomenon*   drug toxicity (e.g., quinidine, tricyclic
irritable tissue (as with MI)   antidepressants)
hypoxia   CHF
digitalis intoxication   stress
(see p. 186)   exercise
electrolyte imbalance (especially hypokalemia and hypocalcemia)
chronic heart disease (ischemic or hypertensive or both)

Treatment only very symptomatic PVCs require treatment

    1. beta blockers (e.g., propranolol) are used for benign and prognostically important (i.e., more frequent and associated with cardiac disease) PVCs[†]

    2. lidocaine or procainamide is administered intravenously for symptomatic PVCs associated with MI or cardiac surgery[†]

KEY POINTS Infrequent PVCs in people with normal hearts are of no concern. In people with heart disease, however, PVCs confer a significant risk of subsequent cardiac death. PVCs are more likely to be symptomatic and need treatment when

    1. there are more than 6/min

    2. they are multiform

    3. there are two or more in a row

    4. there is bigeminy*

    5. there is an R-on-T phenomenon (PVC falling on T wave of preceding beat)

---

*Refer to glossary for more information.

[†]For more information on drug therapy, refer to drug section.

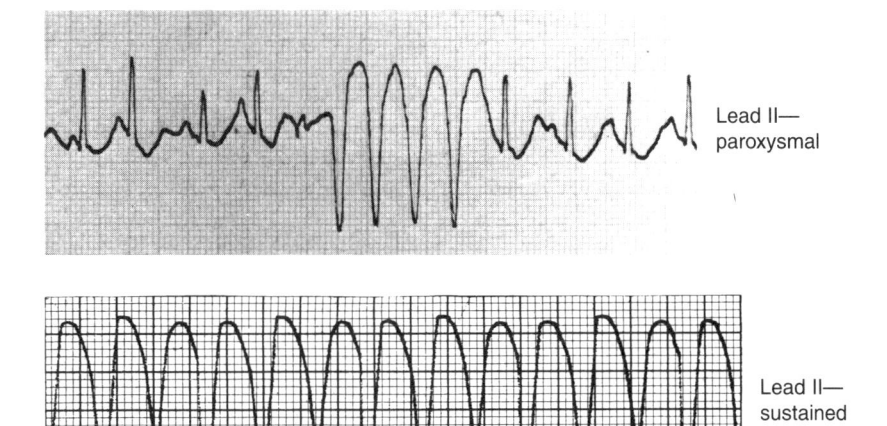

Lead II—
paroxysmal

Lead II—
sustained

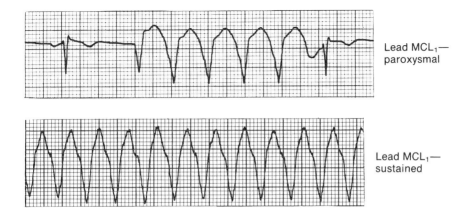

Lead MCL₁—
paroxysmal

Lead MCL₁—
sustained

Continued on following page

V-tach consists of three or more PVCs in a row at a rate >100 bpm.

P Waves similar; AV dissociation* is present during V-tach
Rhythm ventricular, regular
Rate >100 bpm, usually 140 to 200 bpm (ventricular)
QRS >0.12 s and bizarre configuration

Possible Causes acute MI
chronic ischemic heart disease
electrolyte imbalance (especially hypokalemia)
CHF
valvular disease
hypoxia

Treatment 1. precordial thump (only in witnessed arrest when defibrillator and pacemaker are
immediately available)
2. *patient stable:* lidocaine 1 to 1.5 mg/kg body weight IV bolus at 50 mg/min†
3. *patient unstable:* cardioversion* and then drug therapy†
(See Ventricular Tachycardia Algorithm [p. 124] for continued therapy.)
4. Some physicians also give magnesium sulfate as part of the treatment.

See pages 182 to 185 to help differentiate V-tach from SVT with aberrancy.

KEY POINTS • The stability of the patient is based on level of consciousness and vital signs (specifically heart rate and BP); that is, a stable patient is one who remains alert with adequate BP even though rhythm is V-tach.
• The hemodynamic effects of V-tach depend on the rate and presence of myocardial dysfunction (e.g., ischemia or infarction).
• Oftentimes with sustained V-tach a patient becomes unstable (i.e., unconscious or hypotensive or both), requiring cardioversion to convert from V-tach.

---

*Refer to glossary for more information.
†For more information on drug therapy, refer to drug section.

◤ Torsades de Pointes

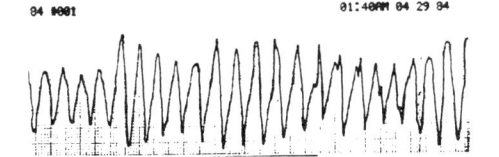

84 #001   01:40AM 04 29 84

Torsades is a type of V-tach characterized by the "twisting" of the QRS around the baseline.

P Waves AV dissociation* is present; P waves usually not seen
Rhythm ventricular, usually irregular
Rate usually >200 bpm
QRS >0.12 s; complexes may have varying heights and appear to rotate around the baseline
QT of basic rhythm should be monitored for lengthening; notify physician if it does

Possible Causes associated with long QT syndrome
        antiarrhythmic therapy (e.g., quinidine, procainamide, disopyramide, bretylium,
          amiodarone, and ibutilide fumarate)
        psychotropic agents (e.g., phenothiazines and tricyclic antidepressants)
        electrolyte imbalances (especially low serum potassium, calcium, or magnesium
          levels)

myocarditis and ischemia or infarct
marked bradycardia
mitral valve prolapse

Treatment 1. initial "treatment" is prevention (e.g., monitoring for lengthening of QT interval)
2. discontinue offending medications (may try antiarrhythmics that do not prolong QT interval)
3. replace electrolytes if necessary; many physicians will order magnesium sulfate IV even with normal serum magnesium levels
4. one may try to "overdrive" the tachycardia with isoproterenol or pacing, but be absolutely sure the rhythm is torsades and *not* sustained V-tach before using isoproterenol, since it could cause intractable V-tach and death[†]
(See Ventricular Tachycardia Algorithm [p. 124] for continued therapy.)

---

*Refer to glossary for more information.
[†]For more information on drug therapy, refer to drug section.

◤ Ventricular Fibrillation (V-Fib)

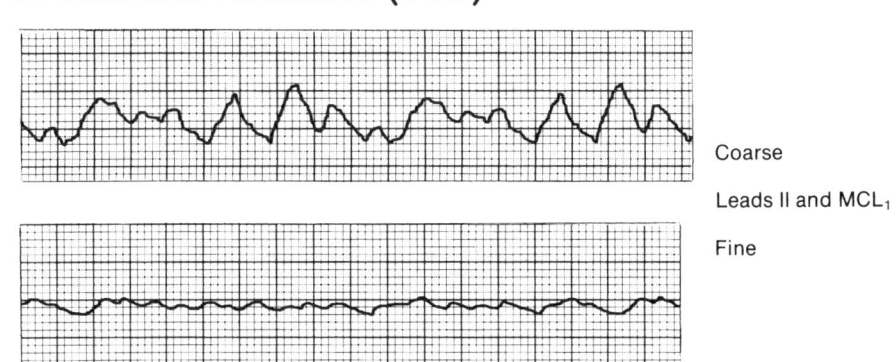

Coarse

Leads II and MCL₁

Fine

V-fib is a lethal dysrhythmia* if not immediately treated!

No organized depolarization,* so *no* contraction. Patient will be unresponsive with no palpable pulse; check ECG leads if otherwise.

Probable Cause reentry phenomenon*

Treatment 1. *immediate* defibrillation* at 200 J
2. initiate cardiac arrest procedure
(See Ventricular Fibrillation Algorithm [p. 122] for continued therapy.)

KEY POINTS "Coarse" and "fine" describe the amplitude of the waves:
- coarse usually means recent onset
- fine usually means V-fib of longer duration

---

*Refer to glossary for more information.

Asystole

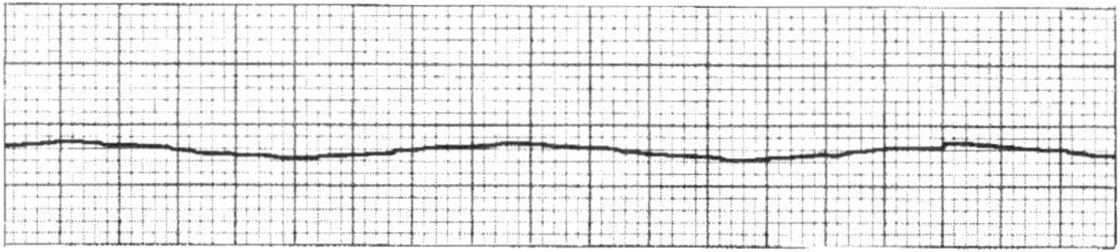

Asystole

Leads II and MCL_1

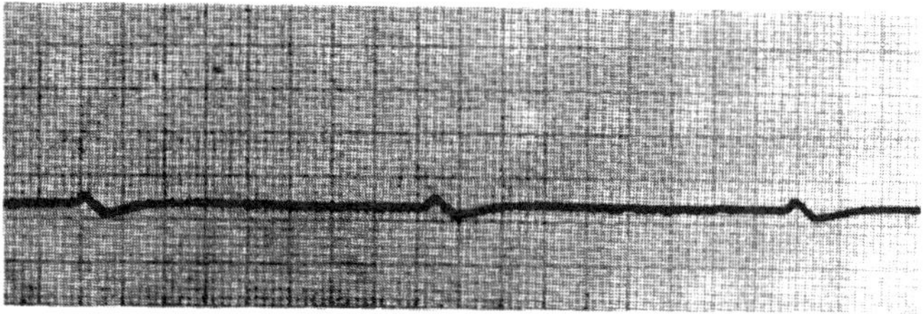

Ventricular standstill

Asystole is also known as "straight line."

*Asystole is a lethal dysrhythmia** if not treated immediately.

Characterized by the absence of any ventricular activity (there may be P waves, in which case the dysrhythmia is called "ventricular standstill").

Treatment   1. initiate cardiopulmonary resuscitation (CPR)
2. initiate cardiac arrest procedure
3. epinephrine 1:10,000 solution 1 mg IV push[†]
(See Asystole Algorithm [p. 130] for continued therapy.)

---

*Refer to glossary for more information.
[†]For more information on drug therapy, refer to drug section.

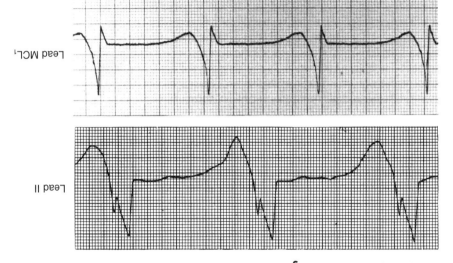

Lead MCL₁

Lead II

P Waves none
Rhythm may be regular or irregular (ventricular)
Rate 20 to 40 bpm (ventricular)
QRS >0.12 s

Possible Causes acute MI   severe hyperkalemia
                      hypoxia   complete AV block
                      acidosis   emergence from cardiac arrest

Treatment 1. epinephrine IV push*
               2. CPR if patient is pulseless

KEY POINT Usually seen only in a cardiac arrest situation.

---

*For more information on drug therapy, refer to drug section.

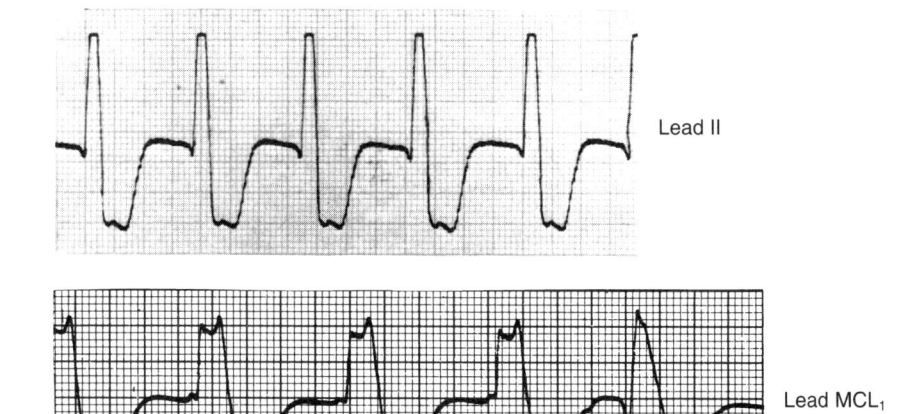

Lead II

Lead MCL₁

P Waves present with AV dissociation* but may be buried within the QRS
Rhythm regular (ventricular)
Rate 40 to 100 bpm (ventricular)
QRS >0.12 s

Possible Causes thought to be an accelerated ventricular escape rhythm,* usually without consequence
common after MI (especially inferior wall)
digitalis toxicity (see p. 186)
reperfusion after thrombolytic therapy*

Treatment usually none required because ventricular rhythm often alternates with NSR at a similar rate
1. if rate > 100 bpm, treat like V-tach (i.e., lidocaine 1 mg/kg body weight at 50 mg/min)†
2. if rate < 60 bpm and patient is symptomatic (i.e., hypotensive, dizzy, or with cool and clammy skin), atropine 0.5 mg IV push can be given†

---

*Refer to glossary for more information.
†For more information on drug therapy, refer to drug section.

First-Degree AV Block

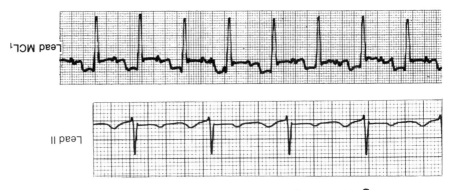

Lead MCL₁

Lead II

P Waves similar, 1:1 with QRS

Rhythm atrial, regular
ventricular, regular

Rate atrial, usually 60 to 100 bpm $\left.\right\}$ same rate
ventricular, usually 60 to 100 bpm

PR >0.20 s and usually consistent

QRS 0.04 to 0.10 s

QT 0.32 to 0.44 s

Possible Causes disease of conduction system
may occur after administration of digitalis or quinidine

Treatment 1. none except to observe for worsening block
2. possibly hold digitalis*

KEY POINT Block occurs at the level of the AV node usually and delays impulses through to ventricles.

---

*For more information on drug therapy, refer to drug section.

◣ Second-Degree AV Block, Mobitz I (Wenckebach)

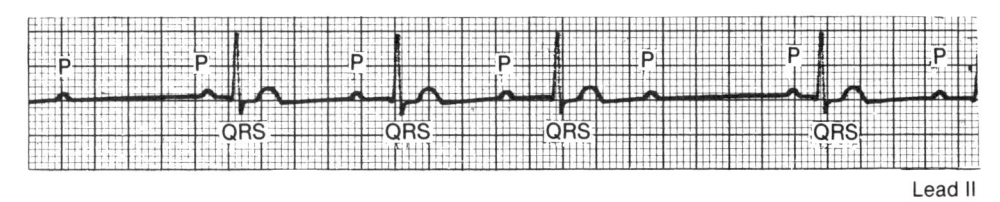

Lead II

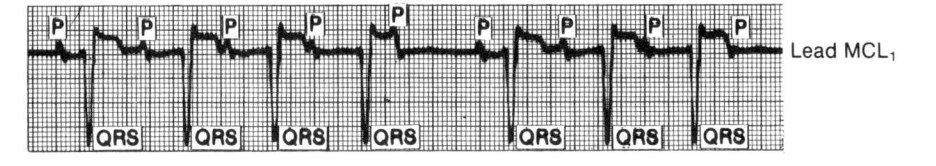

Lead MCL₁

P Waves similar; more Ps than QRSs
Rhythm atrial, regular
       ventricular, irregular (occur in "groups")
Rate atrial > ventricular

PR gradually increases until one QRS is "blocked"; is a cyclic pattern (e.g., PR of 0.20, 0.24, 0.26 s, none; then same sequence is repeated)

QRS 0.04 to 0.10 s

QT 0.32 to 0.44 s

Possible Causes drug effect (e.g., digitalis, propranolol, quinidine, procainamide)
increased parasympathetic tone (vagal stimulation)
after acute MI (usually inferior)

Treatment 1. none unless ventricular rate is slow enough to warrant atropine*
2. observe for worsening block
(See Bradycardia Algorithm [p. 132] for continued therapy.)

---

*For more information on drug therapy, refer to drug section.

Continued on following page

KEY POINTS
- The block occurs at the level of the AV node and is usually transient.
- The "cycles" are referred to according to atrial and ventricular conduction; that is, 4:3 conduction, 3:2 conduction, and so on. The ratio may vary or remain constant.* When 2:1 conduction occurs, it is extremely difficult to differentiate Mobitz I from Mobitz II.†

---

*Refer to glossary for more information.
†Refer to page 92 for help with differentiating blocks.

■ Second-Degree AV Block, Mobitz II

Lead II

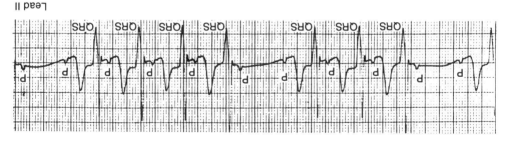

Lead MCL₁

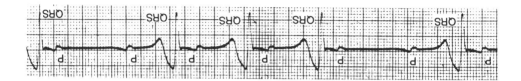

P Waves similar, more Ps than QRSs

Rhythm atrial, regular

ventricular, irregular, unless conduction ratio* is constant

Rate atrial > ventricular

PR constant for conducted beats; may be normal or prolonged (>0.20 s)

QRS may be normal but frequently > 0.10 s

QT usually 0.32 to 0.44 s

Possible Causes acute MI (usually anterior)   hypoxia
chronic ischemic or hypertensive heart   following cardiac surgery
disease or both

Treatment 1. atropine 0.5 mg IV push if patient symptomatic (i.e., dizzy, hypotensive, cool and
clammy skin)†
2. temporary or permanent pacemaker may be indicated
3. observe for worsening block or hemodynamic instability
(See Bradycardia Algorithm [p. 132] for continued therapy.)

---

*Refer to glossary for more information.

†For more information on drug therapy, refer to drug section.

Continued on following page

KEY POINTS
- Block occurs most often at the level of the bundle branches and is associated with an organic lesion in the conduction pathway; it is not a result of drugs or increased parasympathetic tone.
- When 2:1 conduction occurs, it is extremely difficult to differentiate Mobitz I from Mobitz II.*
- Associated with poor prognosis, since progression to third-degree AV block is anticipated.

---

*Refer to page 92 for help with differentiating blocks.

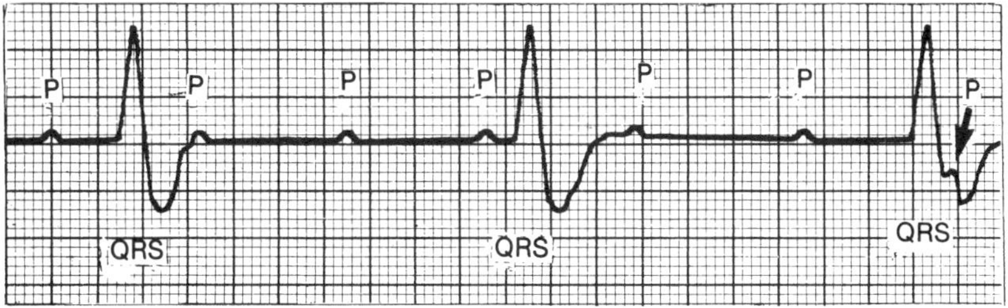

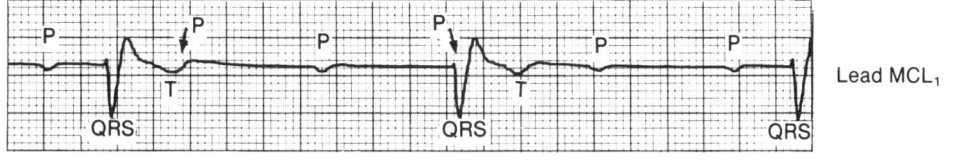

Lead II

Lead MCL₁

P Waves similar, more Ps than QRSs
Rhythm atrial and ventricular both regular
Rate atrial, usually 60 to 100 bpm
        ventricular, 40 to 60 bpm with AV junctional escape rhythm
                    <40 bpm with ventricular escape rhythm
PR varies beat to beat
QRS usually >0.10 s
QT may be normal or long (>0.44 s)

Possible Causes extensive MI (usually anterior)
                extensive ventricular conduction
                    system disease (e.g., fibrosis)
                digitalis intoxication (see p. 186)
                acidosis

cardiac trauma or following
    cardiac surgery
hypoxia
hyperkalemia

Continued on following page

◣ Third-Degree (Complete) AV Block *(Continued)*

Treatment 1. atropine or isoproterenol or both until temporary pacemaker is inserted*
           2. transthoracic pacing may be used until temporary pacemaker inserted
           3. permanent pacemaker indicated
           (See Bradycardia Algorithm [p. 132] for continued therapy.)

KEY POINTS The block can occur either at the level of the AV node or below it (i.e., bundle branches). Complete block at the level of the AV node tends to be transient, whereas complete block at the infranodal level usually tends to be chronic.†

---

*For more information on drug therapy, refer to drug section.
†Refer to page 92 for help with differentiating blocks.

A simple way to determine what type of AV block, if any, is present involves looking at the P waves in relation to QRS complexes and at the PR intervals. Some practitioners also consider the atrial and ventricular rhythms and the QRS width; these can be helpful but are not necessary for diagnosis of an AV block.

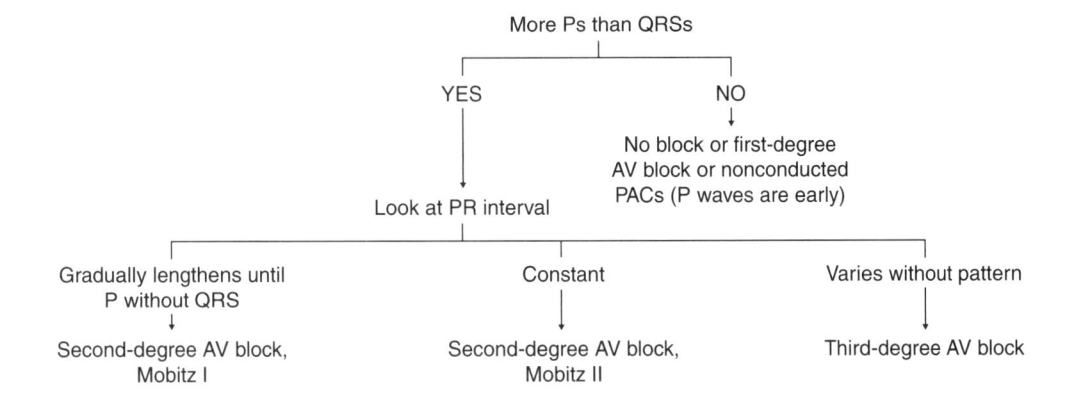

◼ AV Dissociation

"AV dissociation" is a term indicating that the atria and ventricles are being paced independently. Three situations are marked by AV dissociation:
   1. slowing of the rate of the primary pacemaker, as in accelerated idioventricular rhythm
   2. acceleration of the rate of a lower pacemaker, as in ventricular tachycardia
   3. complete AV block

Possible Causes   increased vagal tone
   digitalis toxicity (see p. 186)
   chronic ischemic heart disease
   rheumatic fever

Treatment   based on the type of AV dissociation
   1. increase the rate of the primary pacemaker (e.g., in the setting of accelerated idioventricular rhythm)
   2. decrease the rapid rate of the lower pacemaker (e.g., in the setting of ventricular tachycardia)
   3. atropine may be used until temporary pacemaker is inserted (e.g., in the setting of third-degree AV block)

Mechanisms of action for both catecholamines and antiarrhythmic medications are discussed. Only emergency uses are given for the medications in this section, although some of the drugs are given on a daily basis. When appropriate, the doses given are according to American Heart Association (AHA) Advanced Cardiac Life Support (ACLS) protocols, as known at the time of this printing.

adenosine (Adenocard)
amrinone (Inocor)
atropine
bretylium (Bretylol)
calcium chloride
digoxin (Lanoxin)
diltiazem (Cardizem)
dl-sotalol (Betapace)
dobutamine (Dobutrex)
dopamine (Intropin)
epinephrine (Adrenalin)

ibutilide fumarate (Corvert)
isoproterenol (Isuprel)
lidocaine
magnesium sulfate
morphine
procainamide (Pronestyl, Procan SR)
propranolol (Inderal)
quinidine
sodium bicarbonate
verapamil (Calan, Isoptin)

MECHANISM OF ACTION: CATECHOLAMINES

Catecholamines can be naturally occurring (e.g., norepinephrine, epinephrine, dopamine) or synthetic (e.g., isoproterenol, dobutamine) substances that stimulate specific receptors within the cardiovascular and respiratory systems. The receptors are classified as alpha (α) or beta (β); beta receptors are further divided into β_1 and β_2.

Class	Receptor Location	Results of Stimulation	To Remember
Alpha	Blood vessels	Vasoconstriction	**A**lpha—**A**rteries
Beta$_1$	Heart	Greater contractility Accelerated heart rate	 (β_1—1 heart)
Beta$_2$	Blood vessels Bronchi	Vasodilation Bronchodilation	 (β_2—2 lungs)

MECHANISM OF ACTION: ANTIARRHYTHMIC MEDICATIONS

CORRELATION OF CARDIAC ACTION POTENTIAL PHASES WITH ECG COMPLEXES (REPRESENTS AN "ECG" OF A MYOCARDIAL CELL*)

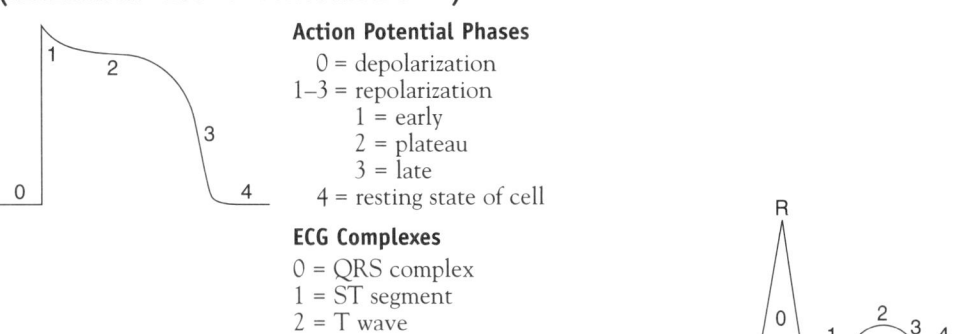

Action Potential Phases

0 = depolarization
1–3 = repolarization
    1 = early
    2 = plateau
    3 = late
4 = resting state of cell

ECG Complexes

0 = QRS complex
1 = ST segment
2 = T wave
3 = late T wave
4 = end of T wave to next QRS complex

---

*This particular action potential is of a Purkinje fiber cell.

Class	Action	Examples
I	Sodium channel blocker	
IA	Moderate phase 0 depression Slows conduction in phase 2 (prolongs repolarization)	Procainamide,* quinidine,* disopyramide, moricizine
IB	Slows conduction in phase 0–1 Shortens repolarization	Lidocaine,* mexiletine, tocainide
IC†	Marked depression in phase 0 (slows depolarization) Slows conduction in phase 4 Little effect on repolarization	Flecainide, propafenone
II	Beta blocker	Propranolol,* acebutolol
III	Prolongs repolarization	Amiodarone, bretylium,* dl-sotalol*
IV	Calcium channel blocker	Verapamil,* diltiazem*

*Discussed further in the medication section.
†Because of their proarrhythmia potential, these drugs are indicated only for life-threatening ventricular arrhythmias when other drugs have failed.

ADENOSINE (ADENOCARD)

Uses   treatment of PSVT

Dose   6 mg rapid IV push (over 1 to 3 s); may be repeated with 12 mg dose in 2 minutes if needed

Side Effects   flushing, dyspnea, and chest pain (common but transient since the half-life of adenosine is less than 5 seconds)

Precautions   1. patients taking theophylline are less sensitive to adenosine and may require larger doses

        2. transient bradycardia, pauses, and ventricular ectopy* are common after termination of PSVT

        3. PSVT may recur because of the short half-life of adenosine

---

*Refer to glossary for more information.

AMRINONE (INOCOR)

Uses short-term treatment of CHF (increases contractility and causes peripheral vasodilation)

Dose initial IV bolus of 0.75 mg/kg body weight given over 2 to 3 minutes; followed by infusion of 5 to 15 µg/kg/min (a common mixture is 200 mg in 40 ml normal saline [NS])

Side Effects angina, increased ventricular ectopy,* hypotension (rare)

Precautions 1. mix only in NS or 0.45% NS solutions
2. optimal use requires hemodynamic monitoring
3. do not use with severe aortic or pulmonic valvular disease

---

*Refer to glossary for more information.

ATROPINE

Uses treatment of symptomatic bradydysrhythmias* (i.e., heart rate <60 bpm and systolic BP <90 mm Hg, with dizziness, cool and clammy skin) by increasing heart rate and improving AV conduction

treatment of asystole and slow pulseless electrical activity (PEA)

Dose *bradycardia:* 0.5 to 1 mg IV push rapidly; may repeat every 3 to 5 minutes up to 3 mg (0.04 mg/kg) total dose

asystole or PEA: 1 mg IV push rapidly; may repeat every 3 to 5 minutes up to 3 mg total dose

atropine may also be given via endotracheal tube, but use 2 to 2.5 times the peripheral dose

Side Effects dry mouth, inability to void, PVCs, pupils dilated, tachycardia

Contraindications glaucoma; use with extreme caution in acute MI

---

*Refer to glossary for more information.

BRETYLIUM (BRETYLOL)

Class III

Uses treatment of V-fib and V-tach not responsive to lidocaine, defibrillation, and epinephrine

Dose *V-fib*: 5 mg/kg IV push; increase to 10 mg/kg and repeat every 5 minutes as needed; total dose not to exceed 35 mg/kg

V-tach: 5 to 10 mg/kg IV over 8 to 10 minutes (may be diluted in 50 ml D$_5$W or NS); may be followed by IV drip at 1 to 2 mg/min (common mixture is 2 g/500 ml D$_5$W or NS, which gives 4 mg/ml)

Side Effects nausea and vomiting from too rapid IV push; syncope; hypotension (sometimes marked)

Precautions 1. keep patient supine (postural hypotension almost always develops)
2. will potentiate catecholamines (e.g., dopamine, epinephrine)
3. not recommended for *prevention* of dysrhythmias* in patient with recent MI

---

*Refer to glossary for more information.

CALCIUM CHLORIDE

Uses treatment of decreased contractility in cardiac arrest only in the presence of hyperkalemia, hypocalcemia, or calcium channel blocker toxicity

Dose 2 to 4 mg/kg of 10% solution IV over 1 to 2 minutes; may repeat every 10 minutes as necessary

Side Effects cardiac arrest with too rapid injection; potentiates digitalis toxicity

Contraindications V-fib because it causes refractory V-fib; *do not* mix with sodium bicarbonate (mixture causes a solid precipitate to form)

Precautions be sure IV is patent; extravasation can cause severe necrosis and sloughing

DIGOXIN (LANOXIN)

Uses to increase myocardial contraction (and thus increase cardiac output) in CHF and cardiogenic shock

to slow heart rate in atrial tachydysrhythmias*

Dose patient is digitalized over 24 hours (total of 1 mg in divided doses); may be given either intravenously or by mouth; maintenance dose is usually given daily or every other day

Side Effects dysrhythmias* (first ECG signs: ST sagging and PR prolonged), yellow vision, gastrointestinal disturbances (e.g., anorexia, nausea and vomiting, abdominal pain), headache (See page 186 for digitalis toxicity.)

Incompatibilities calcium preparations, sodium bicarbonate (flush IV line well between injections of digoxin and these drugs)

Precautions 1. does not control heart rate well during exercise
2. many drug interactions are possible; refer to a medication resource as needed

---

*Refer to glossary for more information.

DILTIAZEM (CARDIZEM LYO-JECT)

Class IV

Uses to decrease ventricular rate in atrial fibrillation or flutter
to convert PSVT to sinus rhythm

Dose IV *push:* 0.25 mg/kg
IV *infusion:* 10 mg/h for up to 24 hours; do not exceed 15 mg/h *or* longer than 24 hours

Side Effects hypotension, site reaction, flushing, dysrhythmias (e.g., bradycardia, AV block)

Contraindications sick sinus syndrome, second- or third-degree AV block in absence of a pacemaker, systolic BP < 90 mm Hg, acute MI

Precautions 1. additive effects on AV node when used with digoxin or beta blockers
2. use with caution in CHF

dl-SOTALOL (BETAPACE)

Class III

Uses treatment of *life-threatening* ventricular dysrhythmias* (e.g., sustained V-tach)

Dose start at 80 mg PO twice daily; dose usually titrated every 2 to 3 days; take on an empty stomach to enhance absorption

Side Effects new ventricular dysrhythmia,* bradycardia, CHF, dizziness, fatigue

Contraindications bradycardia, second- or third-degree AV block, cardiogenic shock, asthma, COPD, congenital or acquired long QT syndromes

Precautions 1. dose is reduced in patients with renal impairment
2. may be proarrhythmic; torsades de pointes has occurred
3. use with extreme caution in sick sinus syndrome

---

*Refer to glossary for more information.

DOBUTAMINE (DOBUTREX)

Class catecholamine

Use short-term treatment of cardiogenic shock or heart failure or both

Dose 250 mg/250 ml D_5W or NS; start at 2.5 to 10 µg/kg/min and titrate according to patient's response; may use up to 40 µg/kg/min; optimal use requires hemodynamic monitoring

Side Effects increased heart rate, PVCs, angina, hypertension, headache

Incompatibilities sodium bicarbonate (do not give bicarbonate in dobutamine IV line if possible; if unavoidable, flush line well before and after)

Precautions 1. may markedly increase heart rate or systolic BP or both
2. may cause or worsen ventricular ectopy*
3. tricyclic antidepressants may increase the risk of hypertension

---

*Refer to glossary for more information.

DOPAMINE (INTROPIN)

Class catecholamine

Uses treatment of hypotension in CHF or cardiogenic shock
treatment of traumatic or septic shock
to increase perfusion to kidneys (low dose)

Dose 400 to 800 mg in 500 ml D_5W or NS; usually titrated to keep systolic BP >90 to 100 mm Hg; start at 2.5 to 5 µg/kg/min and increase as needed; if titrated beyond 20 µg/kg/min, renal perfusion is sacrificed

Side Effects elevated BP, palpitations, tachycardia, bradycardia, angina, azotemia, vasoconstriction, headache

Contraindications tachydysrhythmias,* V-fib, pheochromocytoma

Precautions 1. be sure IV line is patent (can cause tissue necrosis)
2. correct hypovolemia before beginning dopamine infusion
3. monitor BP frequently (every 2 to 5 minutes) until stabilized at desired level
4. therapy should be titrated gradually

Incompatibilities sodium bicarbonate (do not give bicarbonate in dopamine IV line if possible; if unavoidable, flush line well before and after) because dopamine is inactivated by alkaline solutions

---

*Refer to glossary for more information.

EPINEPHRINE (ADRENALIN)

Class catecholamine

Uses improvement of myocardial and central nervous system (CNS) blood flow during CPR
to initiate spontaneous contraction in cardiac arrest
to elevate BP in patient not in cardiac arrest

Dose 1 mg (10 ml of 1:10,000 solution) IV push every 3 to 5 minutes; may give 2 to 2.5 mg via endotracheal tube
alternative dosing (if 1 mg dose has failed):
• 1 mg, 3 mg, and 5 mg IV boluses given 3 minutes apart
• IV boluses of 2 to 5 mg given every 3 to 5 minutes
IV infusion may be administered, starting at 1 μg/kg and titrated to optimum hemodynamic effect (usually 2 to 10 μg/kg); common mixture is 1 mg in 500 ml D$_5$W or NS

Side Effects anxiety, angina, headache, PVCs, V-tach

Contraindications hyperthyroidism, hypertension, collapse due to phenothiazine overdose (may further lower BP)

Precautions **1.** give *very* cautiously with isoproterenol (both are direct cardiac stimulants)
2. inactivated by alkaline solutions (be especially careful to flush IV line between injections of sodium bicarbonate and epinephrine)
3. use with extreme caution in patients with longstanding bronchial asthma or emphysema
4. tricyclic antidepressants may increase the risk of hypertension
5. give only 1:10,000 solution IV (administration of 1:1000 solution IV can result in severe hypertension and cerebral hemorrhage)
6. extravasation can lead to necrosis of tissue; IV infusion should be given only via central line

IBUTILIDE FUMARATE (CORVERT)

Class III

Uses rapid conversion of recent onset atrial fibrillation or flutter

Dose initial IV infusion given over 10 minutes (dose as designated below); may repeat 10 minutes after initial infusion if dysrhythmia* has not stopped; may administer undiluted or mixed in 50 ml D_5W or NS

≥ 60 kg body weight: 1 mg (one vial)

< 60 kg body weight: 0.01 mg/kg

Side Effects polymorphic ventricular tachycardia (torsades de pointes) may occur, usually presenting within first hour after ibutilide fumarate infusion; PVCs, headache, hypotension, bundle branch block, AV block

Precautions 1. can cause life-threatening dysrhythmias (e.g., torsades de pointes), especially in patients with history of CHF; observe patients with continuous ECG monitoring for at least 4 hours following infusion

2. patients with A-fib of at least 2 days duration must be anticoagulated for at least 2 weeks before ibutilide fumarate can be used

3. do not give other class III or IA antiarrhythmics within 4 hours of infusion of ibutilide fumarate

---

*Refer to glossary for more information.

ISOPROTERENOL (ISUPREL)

Class catecholamine

Uses treatment of hemodynamically significant bradycardias in the denervated hearts of heart transplant patients or refractory torsades de pointes (only as a temporary measure until pacemaker therapy is initiated)

Dose 1 mg/250 ml D_5W, which gives 4 µg/ml; titrate to keep heart rate at 60 to 100 bpm; usual dose is 2 to 10 µg/min

Side Effects *tachycardia*, V-tach, PVCs, V-fib, hypotension, headache, angina, flushing

Contraindications tachycardia, cardiac arrest, hypotension

Precautions 1. give *very* cautiously with epinephrine (both are direct cardiac stimulants)
2. use with extreme caution in patients with recent MI
3. use with extreme caution, if at all, to treat symptomatic bradycardia
4. tricyclic antidepressants may increase the risk of hypertension

LIDOCAINE

Class IB

Uses treatment of PVCs, V-tach, V-fib, and wide-QRS tachycardias of uncertain origin

Dose 1 to 1.5 mg/kg IV bolus at 50 mg/min; may repeat 0.5 to 1.5 mg/kg every 5 to 10 minutes up to total dose of 3 mg/kg; follow with drip at 1 to 4 mg/min

If lidocaine is being given prophylactically, 0.5 mg/kg boluses should be given to total dose of only 2 mg/kg (unless ectopy persists)

2 g/500 ml D$_5$W: 1 mg = 15 microdrops

Side Effects (transient) drowsiness, numbness, tingling, blurred vision, ringing in ears, agitation, dizziness, slurred speech

Overdose anaphylaxis, hypotension, twitching, convulsions, coma, cardiovascular collapse

Contraindications heart rate <60 bpm; *do not* use with any kind of AV block; use cautiously in patients with severe liver disease or renal failure or who are over 70 years old

MAGNESIUM SULFATE

Uses   treatment of choice for torsades de pointes
to reduce incidence of postinfarction ventricular dysrhythmias*

Dose   *V-fib or V-tach:* 1 to 2 g in 100 ml D$_5$W, given over 1 to 2 minutes
postinfarction dysrhythmias: 1 to 2 g in 100 ml D$_5$W, given over 5 to 60 minutes; follow with
infusion of 0.5 to 1 g/h for up to 24 hours

Side Effects   hypotension, sweating, drowsiness, flushing, muscle weakness

Precautions   1. observe for, and report to physician, any side effects
2. give cautiously with AV block or impaired renal function

---

*Refer to glossary for more information.

MORPHINE

Uses relief of severe pain and apprehension
treatment of pulmonary edema (causes venous dilation, which decreases the amount of blood returning to the heart and thus to the lungs)

Dose 2 to 5 mg increments, usually up to 10 to 15 mg total; usually may be repeated every 2 to 3 hours as needed (PRN)

Side Effects orthostatic hypotension, slight respiratory depression, increased intracranial pressure, lightheadedness, sedation, disorientation

Overdose severe respiratory depression and hypotension, coma, pinpoint pupils, death; overdose can be treated with administration of naloxone (Narcan)

PROCAINAMIDE (PRONESTYL, PROCAN SR)

Class IA

Uses treatment of PVCs and recurrent V-tach when lidocaine has failed or is contraindicated
treatment of supraventricular dysrhythmias* (as with quinidine) or wide-QRS PSVT of uncertain origin

Dose IV: 20 to 30 mg/min until QRS widens by 50%, hypotension develops, or dysrhythmia is suppressed; total dose not to exceed 17 mg/kg; follow either with 1 to 4 mg/min IV drip or PO; IV drip: 2 g/500 ml D_5W: 1 mg = 15 microdrops

PO: 250 to 750 mg every 3 to 6 hours *or* sustained release up to 50 mg/kg/d given in divided doses 12 hours apart

Side Effects *minor:* nausea and vomiting, weakness, confusion, giddiness

major: severe hypotension, QRS widening, QT prolonged, asystole, V-fib, V-tach, 1:1 conduction of atrial flutter (with IV dose), lupuslike syndrome, agranulocytosis (ask about fever or sore throat)

Precautions 1. use with extreme caution in first- and second-degree AV block, digitalis intoxication, V-tach, liver or renal impairment, and after MI
2. avoid using in patients with preexisting QT prolongation, torsades de pointes, or lupus erythematosus

---

*Refer to glossary for more information.

PROPRANOLOL (INDERAL)

Class II

Uses control of ventricular rate in A-fib, atrial flutter, A-tach
suppression of ectopic beats and PSVT
reduction of the extent of nonfatal infarction and recurrent ischemia
treatment of symptomatic benign or prognostically important PVCs

Dose IV: total dose of 0.1 mg/kg at rate not to exceed 1 mg/min
PO: 180 to 320 mg/d given in divided doses

Side Effects bradycardia, cardiac failure, hypoglycemia, cardiac standstill, hypotension,
respiratory distress, vertigo

Contraindications complete AV block, COPD, asthma, CHF, cardiogenic shock

Precautions 1. give IV cautiously; can precipitate hypotension and cardiovascular collapse
2. may trigger irreversible bronchospasm if given to patient with asthma
3. may mask the signs of hypoglycemia in diabetes

QUINIDINE

Class IA

Uses treatment of virtually all dysrhythmias* (but used primarily for supraventricular rhythms)

Dose (highly individualized) PO: 200 to 300 mg every 6 to 8 hours *or* sustained release 300 to 600 mg every 8 to 12 hours

Side Effects *minor:* diarrhea, nausea and vomiting, cramps, fever, headache, vertigo, visual disturbances, thrombocytopenia

major: severe hypotension, syncope, cardiac standstill, increased AV or bundle branch block, tachycardia (especially torsades de pointes)

Contraindications complete AV block, aberrant rhythms* due to escape mechanism, myasthenia gravis, history of long QT syndrome

Precautions 1. use with extreme caution with first- or second-degree AV block, extensive MI, digitalis intoxication, impaired liver or renal function

2. concurrent use with digoxin increases digoxin levels

3. notify physician if QT intervals lengthen

---

*Refer to glossary for more information.

SODIUM BICARBONATE

Use treatment of metabolic acidosis or hyperkalemia; potentially useful in tricyclic antidepressant overdose; no longer routinely recommended for cardiac arrest

Dose 1 mEq/kg IV initially; repeat doses according to arterial blood gas determinations; if blood gas determinations are not available, may use one half of initial dose every 10 minutes

Contraindications metabolic or respiratory alkalosis

Precautions 1. use only after CPR, defibrillation, ventilation, and drug therapy have been tried
2. use with caution in patient with cardiac or liver disease (1 amp = 300 ml NS in salt content)
3. incompatible with any other drug; flush IV line before and after injection
4. may cause metabolic alkalosis

VERAPAMIL (CALAN, ISOPTIN)

Class IV

Uses to enhance conversion of supraventricular tachydysrhythmias* to sinus rhythm temporary control of rapid ventricular rate in A-fib, atrial flutter, or multifocal atrial tachycardia

Dose 2.5 to 5 mg IV over at least 2 minutes; may repeat 5 to 10 mg every 15 to 30 minutes to total dose of 20 mg

Side Effects (Infrequent) symptomatic hypotension (may be greater in elderly), severe tachycardia, bradycardia, CHF

Contraindications hypotension, cardiogenic shock, second- or third-degree AV block, severe CHF (unless due to rapid SVTs treatable with verapamil), sick sinus syndrome

Precautions 1. patients with A-fib or atrial flutter with an accessory pathway (e.g., preexcitation syndromes*) can develop a rapid ventricular rate (e.g., 1:1 conduction in atrial flutter)
2. concurrent use with beta blockers (especially if either or both are given IV) has an additive effect on AV node conduction

---

*Refer to glossary for more information.

The following algorithms are intended as guidelines in the treatment of cardiac arrest. Some patients may require care other than that stated. Each algorithm assumes that the rhythm is continuing in spite of the therapy.

When applicable, CPR continues when there is no pulse. The pulse and rhythm should be rechecked after each defibrillation-cardioversion or after medication is administered.

VENTRICULAR FIBRILLATION—PULSELESS VENTRICULAR TACHYCARDIA

ABCs
↓
CPR until defibrillator available
↓
V-fib or V-tach present on defibrillator
↓
Defibrillate up to 3 times, at 200 J,
200–300 J, and 360 J, if needed for
persistent V-fib or V-tach
↓
Continue CPR
↓
Intubate; give 100% O_2; check for
adequate breath sounds bilaterally
↓
Obtain IV access
↓
Epinephrine 1 mg IV push*
(repeat every 3 to 5 minutes)
↓

Defibrillate 360 J within
30 to 60 seconds of epinephrine

↓

Administer medications of probable benefit
- lidocaine 1.5 mg/kg IV push; may repeat
  in 3 to 5 minutes to loading dose of 3 mg/kg
- bretylium 5 mg/kg IV push; may repeat in
  10 minutes at 10 mg/kg
- magnesium sulfate 1 to 2 g IV (in torsades
  de pointes)
- procainamide 30 mg/min to total dose
  of 17 mg/kg
- sodium bicarbonate 1 mEq/kg IV

↓

Defibrillate at 360 J, 30 to 60 seconds after
each dose of medication

NOTE With return of spontaneous circulation,
- assess vital signs
- support airway and breathing
- provide medications appropriate for blood pressure, heart rate, and rhythm

---

*See page 108 for alternative dosing suggestions.

VENTRICULAR TACHYCARDIA/WIDE-QRS TACHYCARDIA

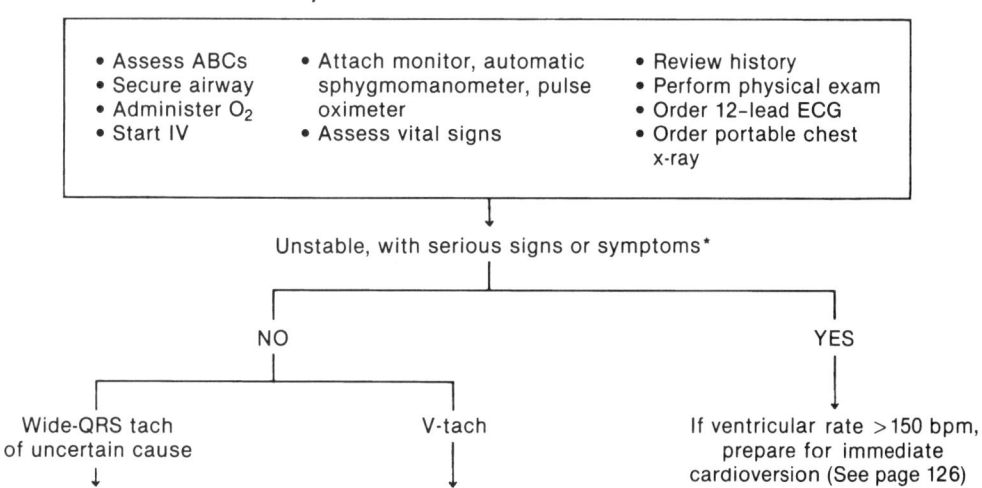

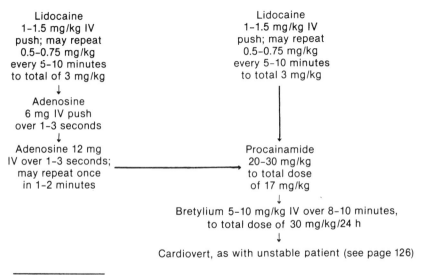

Lidocaine
1–1.5 mg/kg IV
push; may repeat
0.5–0.75 mg/kg
every 5–10 minutes
to total of 3 mg/kg
↓
Adenosine
6 mg IV push
over 1–3 seconds
↓
Adenosine 12 mg
IV over 1–3 seconds;
may repeat once
in 1–2 minutes

Lidocaine
1–1.5 mg/kg IV
push; may repeat
0.5–0.75 mg/kg
every 5–10 minutes
to total 3 mg/kg
↓
Procainamide
20–30 mg/kg
to total dose
of 17 mg/kg
↓
Bretylium 5–10 mg/kg IV over 8–10 minutes,
to total dose of 30 mg/kg/24 h
↓
Cardiovert, as with unstable patient (see page 126)

---

*Signs and symptoms may include chest pain, shortness of breath, decreased level of consciousness, low blood pressure, shock, CHF, acute MI, and pulmonary congestion.

ELECTRICAL CARDIOVERSION (FOR PATIENT WITH PULSE)

Tachycardia with serious signs and symptoms
related to tachycardia*
↓
If ventricular rate > 150 bpm, prepare for
immediate cardioversion (cardioversion
usually not needed if rate < 150 bpm)
↓
May give brief trial of medications,
based on type of arrhythmia
↓
Check: O$_2$ saturation
suction device
IV line
intubation equipment
↓

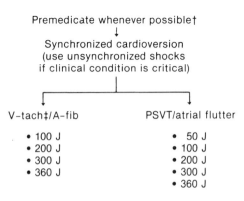

Premedicate whenever possible†
↓
Synchronized cardioversion
(use unsynchronized shocks
if clinical condition is critical)

V-tach‡/A-fib

- 100 J
- 200 J
- 300 J
- 360 J

PSVT/atrial flutter

- 50 J
- 100 J
- 200 J
- 300 J
- 360 J

---

*Signs and symptoms may include chest pain, shortness of breath, decreased level of consciousness, low blood pressure, shock, CHF, acute MI, and pulmonary congestion.

†May be sedative with or without a narcotic.

‡Treat polymorphic V-tach (torsades de pointes) like V-fib.

PULSELESS ELECTRICAL ACTIVITY (PEA)*

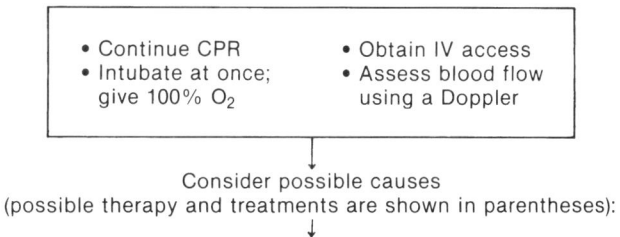

> • Continue CPR
> • Intubate at once; give 100% O_2
> • Obtain IV access
> • Assess blood flow using a Doppler

Consider possible causes
(possible therapy and treatments are shown in parentheses):

↓

- Pulmonary embolus (surgery, thrombolytics)
- Acidosis (bicarb if caused by metabolic acidosis or tricyclic antidepressant overdose)
- Tension pneumothorax (needle decompression)
  Tamponade (pericardiocentesis)
- Hypovolemia (volume infusion)
  Hypoxia (ventilation/oxygenation)
  Hypothermia
  Hyperkalemia (sodium bicarbonate may help)
- Massive acute MI

• Drug overdoses such as tricyclics, digitalis,
beta blockers, or calcium channel blockers
↓
Epinephrine 1 mg IV push; repeat every 3–5 minutes†
↓
If absolute bradycardia (rate <60 bpm) or relative
bradycardia, give atropine 1 mg IV (may repeat every
3 to 5 minutes to total dose of 3 mg)

---

*PEA includes: electromechanical dissociation (EMD), pseudo-EMD, idioventricular rhythms, ventricular escape rhythms, bradyasystolic rhythms, and postdefibrillation idioventricular rhythms.

†See page 108 for alternative dosing suggestions.

ASYSTOLE

- Continue CPR
- Intubate at once; give 100% O_2
- Obtain IV access
- Confirm in second lead

↓

Consider possible causes

- Hypoxia
- Hyperkalemia
- Hypokalemia
- Preexisting acidosis
- Drug overdose
- Hypothermia

↓

Consider immediate transcutaneous pacing

↓

Epinephrine 1 mg IV push, every 3–5 minutes*

↓

Atropine 1 mg IV; repeat every 3–5 minutes
to total dose of 3 mg

↓

Consider termination of efforts

---

* See page 108 for alternative dosing suggestions.

BRADYCARDIA

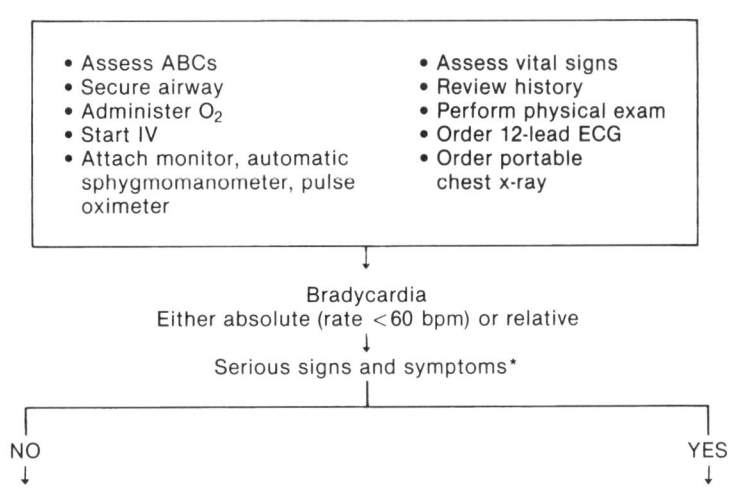

- Assess ABCs
- Secure airway
- Administer O₂
- Start IV
- Attach monitor, automatic sphygmomanometer, pulse oximeter

- Assess vital signs
- Review history
- Perform physical exam
- Order 12-lead ECG
- Order portable chest x-ray

Bradycardia
Either absolute (rate <60 bpm) or relative

Serious signs and symptoms*

NO

YES

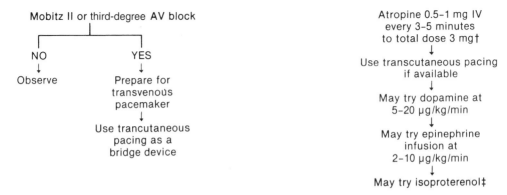

Mobitz II or third-degree AV block

NO → Observe

YES → Prepare for transvenous pacemaker → Use trancutaneous pacing as a bridge device

Atropine 0.5–1 mg IV every 3–5 minutes to total dose 3 mg†
↓
Use transcutaneous pacing if available
↓
May try dopamine at 5–20 µg/kg/min
↓
May try epinephrine infusion at 2–10 µg/kg/min
↓
May try isoproterenol‡

---

*Signs and symptoms must be related to slow rate; they may include chest pain, shortness of breath, decreased level of consciousness, low blood pressure, shock, acute MI, CHF, and pulmonary congestion.

†Denervated transplanted hearts will not respond to atropine. Go at once to pacing, catecholamine infusion, or both.

‡Use with extreme caution if at all.

SUPRAVENTRICULAR TACHYCARDIA

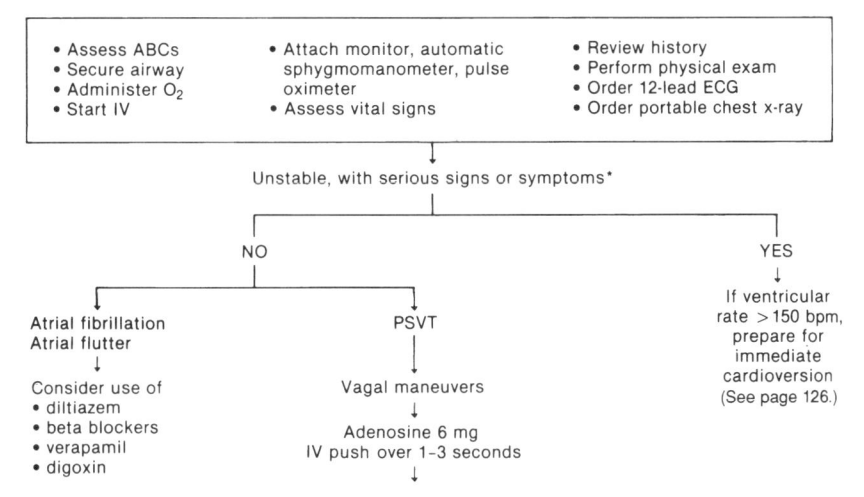

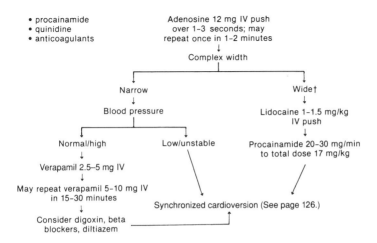

- procainamide
- quinidine
- anticoagulants

Adenosine 12 mg IV push
over 1-3 seconds; may
repeat once in 1-2 minutes
↓
Complex width

Narrow
↓
Blood pressure

Wide†
↓
Lidocaine 1-1.5 mg/kg
IV push
↓
Procainamide 20-30 mg/min
to total dose 17 mg/kg

Normal/high
↓
Verapamil 2.5–5 mg IV
↓
May repeat verapamil 5-10 mg IV
in 15-30 minutes
↓
Consider digoxin, beta
blockers, diltiazem

Low/unstable

Synchronized cardioversion (See page 126.)

---

*Signs and symptoms may include chest pain, shortness of breath, decreased level of consciousness, low blood pressure, shock, CHF, acute MI, and pulmonary congestion.

†If wide-QRS tachycardia is known to be PSVT and BP is not low, verapamil can be given.

135

This section is a review of the 12-lead ECG for diagnosis of ischemia and acute myocardial infarction (MI), including right ventricular infarction. Critical left anterior descending (LAD) artery stenosis (commonly known as Wellens syndrome) will also be discussed. The criteria to determine bundle branch block (BBB) and chamber hypertrophy and to differentiate ventricular ectopy from aberrancy will be given. For further information, refer to the references.

LIMB LEADS

Each of the 12 leads views the heart from a different position, giving a composite picture of what is occurring electrically in the heart. The electrodes used to obtain the 12-lead ECG are right arm (RA), right leg (RL), left arm (LA), left leg (LL), and 6 chest leads.

Leads I, II, and III are called bipolar limb leads because each has a negative and a positive electrode. The right leg lead is the ground lead.

Lead I	(–) right arm	(+) left arm
Lead II	(–) right arm	(+) left leg
Lead III	(–) left arm	(+) left leg

The remaining three limb leads are called "augmented voltage" leads: aVR, aVL, and aVF. They are unipolar because there is one positive electrode and all the remaining limb leads are combined into a ground, which is considered negative. The positive electrodes are as follows:

aVR	right arm
aVL	left arm
aVF	left foot (actually the lead is placed on the left leg)

Continued on following page

PRECORDIAL LEADS

Leads V_1 to V_6 are called precordial (or chest) leads. Each is a unipolar lead. The placement of the electrodes is as follows:

V_1 fourth intercostal space, right sternal border
V_2 fourth intercostal space, left sternal border
V_3 halfway between V_2 and V_4
V_4 fifth intercostal space at midclavicular line
V_5 anterior axillary line directly lateral to V_4
V_6 midaxillary line directly lateral to V_5

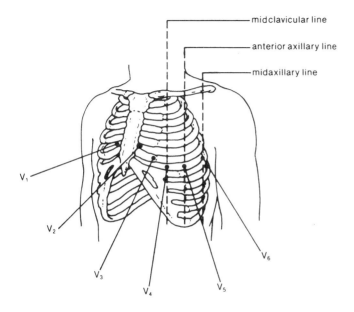

midclavicular line

anterior axillary line

midaxillary line

V_1

V_2

V_3

V_4

V_5

V_6

AXIS DETERMINATION

The mean axis is the predominant direction of the electrical current in the heart; it can be affected by conduction abnormalities, MI, or ventricular hypertrophy. Unless stated otherwise, the term "axis" refers to the axis of the QRS complex. There are many methods for determining the axis; a quick "quadrant method" is discussed here.

Look at leads I and II; determine if the QRS complexes in these leads are predominantly positive (upright) or negative. Because of the electrode placement, lead I "divides" the chest vertically, with the right side being "negative" and the left side "positive." Similarly, lead II divides the chest horizontally, with the upper half being "negative" and the lower half "positive." Thus the following chart can be drawn:

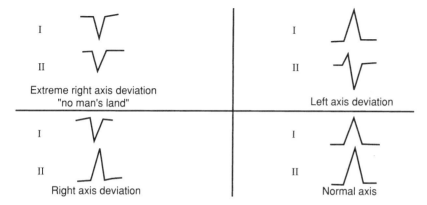

I

II

Extreme right axis deviation
"no man's land"

I

II

Left axis deviation

I

II

Right axis deviation

I

II

Normal axis

NORMAL 12-LEAD ECG

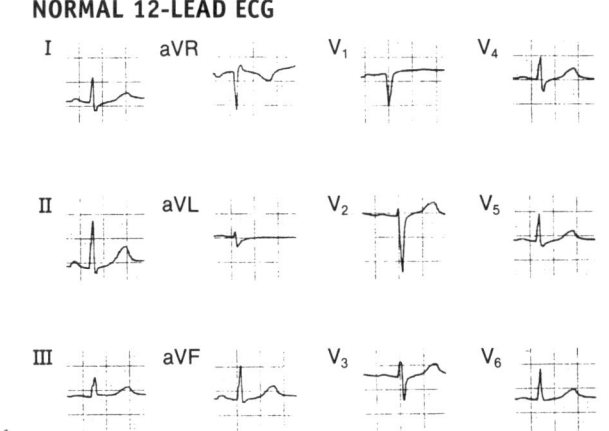

The aVR lead cannot be used to diagnose acute MI but may be used in determining the mean axis. In most people, all complexes are negative in aVR.

Notice that as you look from V_1 to V_6, the R wave becomes taller and the S wave becomes shallower; this is normal R wave progression. The R wave and the S wave should become of equal height, or the R wave should become taller than the S wave in V_3 or V_4. Also notice that all of the ST segments are isoelectric (level with the baseline), and the T waves are upright in all leads except aVR and, in some people, V_1.

RIGHT ATRIAL ABNORMALITY (P PULMONALE)

Cause probably due to increased sympathetic stimulation and position of the diaphragm associated with COPD

Clinical Implications may be associated with congenital heart disease or right ventricular hypertrophy*; aids in evaluation of the severity of COPD

ECG Changes
- P wave duration normal (< 0.11 s)
- tall, peaked P waves in II, III, and aVF (amplitude increases with severity of disease)

---

*Refer to glossary for more information.

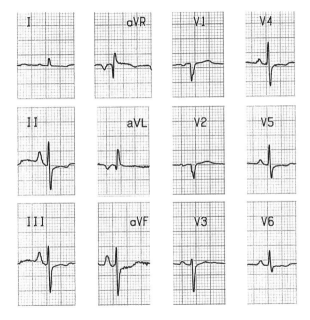

LEFT ATRIAL ABNORMALITY (P MITRALE)

Cause probably associated with conduction defect rather than actual hypertrophy* or dilation

Clinical Implications often present in hypertension; may occur with cardiomyopathy, aortic or mitral valvular disease, and, transiently, with pulmonary edema

ECG Changes • prolonged P wave duration (> 0.12 s)
• notched, upright P wave in I, II, and V_4 through V_6 (like an "m"—to remember, think "m" for "mitral" [valve on left side of heart])
• P wave in V_1 is biphasic with deep negative wave (> 1 mm)
• often accompanied by right ventricular hypertrophy (RVH)

---

*Refer to glossary for more information.

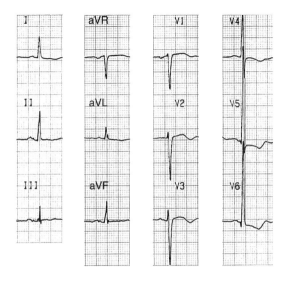

◤ Ventricular Hypertrophy

TYPES

1. Concentric hypertrophy
   - ventricular wall thickens in relation to ventricular cavity size (see p. 149)
   - results from pressure overload related to increased systolic tension (e.g., with hypertension or aortic stenosis)
2. Eccentric hypertrophy
   - chamber dilates; ventricular wall thickness remains relatively normal in relation to chamber size (see p. 149)
   - results from volume overload related to increased end-diastolic wall stress

DIAGNOSTIC TESTS

1. Echocardiogram: superior to ECG for diagnosing mild hypertrophy and for monitoring changes in enlargement
2. Cardiac nuclear studies
3. ECG: does not differentiate between the types of hypertrophy

RA	Right atrium
RV	Right ventricle
LA	Left atrium
LV	Left ventricle

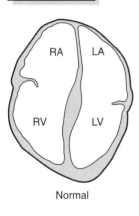

Normal

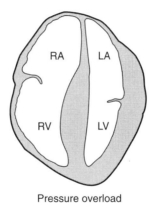

Pressure overload

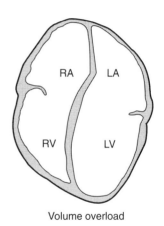

Volume overload

149

RIGHT VENTRICULAR HYPERTROPHY (RVH)

Causes cor pulmonale
cystic fibrosis
COPD
pulmonary fibrosis or primary pulmonary hypertension
congenital pulmonary fibrosis or tetralogy of Fallot

ECG Changes* • right axis deviation +90° to +180° (lead I negative, lead II positive)
• tall R waves in V_1 (R in V_1 > 7 mm; S in V_1 < 2 mm)
• deep S waves in V_4 through V_6 (> 7 mm)
• often accompanied by right atrial abnormality (see p. 144)

---

*Nuclear imaging and echocardiogram are superior in diagnosing RVH.

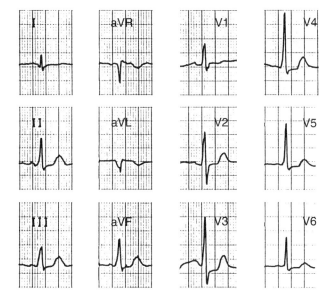

151

LEFT VENTRICULAR HYPERTROPHY (LVH)

Causes aortic stenosis
   chronic systemic hypertension

ECG Changes* (the greater the number of changes the greater the likelihood of LVH):
- S in V_1 plus R in V_5 or V_6 is at least 35 mm
- R in aVL plus S in V_3 > 28 mm (males) or > 20 mm (females)
- ST and T wave depression in I, aVL, V_5, and V_6 (associated with myocardial ischemia)
- left atrial abnormality in V_1 (see p. 146)
- left axis deviation $-30°$ to $-90°$ (lead I positive, lead II negative)
- normal QRS width

---

*ECG signs are not specific; diagnosis may be "clouded" by acute MI, bundle branch block, inaccurate precordial lead placement; echocardiogram is superior in diagnosing LVH.

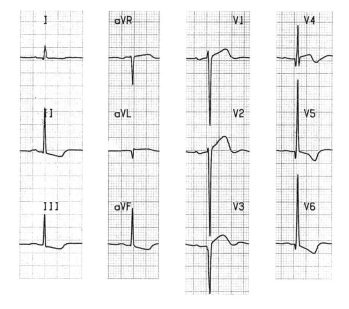

153

Q WAVE MYOCARDIAL INFARCTION

Definition necrosis (or death) of myocardium due to lack of oxygenated blood to the tissue.

Diagnosis of MI is based on patient history, ECG tracings, and laboratory values. *No single ECG is diagnostic*; it needs to be compared with previous tracings to check for changes. The initial ECG can only suggest an MI; successive tracings lead to a positive diagnosis. *No one monitoring lead can diagnose an MI or even ischemia or injury*; although there may be changes, they are not conclusive. Serial 12-lead ECGs are required for diagnosis.

ACUTE ECG CHANGES (ON STANDARDIZED 12-LEAD ECG*)

Although other factors (e.g., drugs or electrolytes) may also cause ECG changes, the changes discussed here are those from hypoxic causes (coronary artery spasm or thrombus).

---

*Refer to glossary for more information.

T wave inversion is a sign of ischemia.

ST depression (>1 mm) and ST elevation (>1 mm) are signs of injury. ST elevation will be seen in affected leads; ST depression will be seen in reciprocal leads or in non-Q-wave MI. (See sections on ECG Changes [p. 156] and Non-Q-Wave Myocardial Infarction [p. 172] for more information.)

Q wave is a sign of necrosis. To be diagnostic of an MI, the Q wave must be *either* equal to or greater than 0.04 second wide or more than one quarter of the total height of the QRS complex.

Early Onset Acute MI T wave inversion
During the Process of a Q Wave MI ST elevation (in affected leads) with reciprocal changes; then T wave inverting, ST returning to baseline, Q wave beginning to develop in affected leads
Old MI ST normal, T wave inverted or upright, Q wave present in affected leads

Q WAVE MYOCARDIAL INFARCTION *(Continued)*

ECG CHANGES

Ischemia, injury, and infarct of the ventricle are reflected in the 12-lead ECG; each area of the ventricle is reflected in certain leads.

		Acute Changes
anterior wall	V_1, V_2, V_3, V_4	ST elevation
inferior wall	II, III, aVF	T wave inversion
lateral wall	I, aVL, V_5, V_6	development of Q wave or loss of R wave

Some practitioners separate anterior leads into septal (V_1 and V_2) and anterior (V_2, V_3, V_4).

		Acute Changes
posterior wall	V_1, V_2	tall R wave
		ST depression
		T wave inversion

More than one area can be involved, e.g., anterolateral wall MI with changes in leads V_1 through V_6.

Reciprocal changes occur in the area opposite that with acute damage (injury or infarct). Reciprocal changes are ST depression and T wave inversion or tall, upright T wave, depending on the stage of the MI. For example, ECG shows acute changes in anterior leads (ST elevation); inferior leads should show reciprocal changes (ST depression and T wave inverted or upright).

Anterior and inferior leads are reciprocal for each other.

Septal and lateral leads are reciprocal for each other.

Q WAVE MYOCARDIAL INFARCTION *(Continued)*

ANTERIOR MYOCARDIAL INFARCTION

Cause blockage of the left main or LAD artery

ECG Changes seen in leads V_1 through V_4
- Initial changes include ST elevation in these leads.
- As the MI progresses, there is loss of R wave progression; that is, QRS complexes in V_1 through V_4 have only small, if any, R waves. (See also section on Normal 12-Lead ECG [p. 142].)

Possible Complications after MI anterior MI is thought to be the most serious of MIs because it is associated with the most complications:

dysrhythmias* (specifically PVCs, V-tach, V-fib)	death (usually due to pump failure or myocardial rupture)
pericarditis	ventricular aneurysm
CHF	papillary muscle dysfunction
cardiogenic shock	

KEY POINT Any AV block associated with anterior MI (e.g., bundle branch block or second- or third-degree block) is often permanent because the LAD artery also supplies the lower conduction system.

---

*Refer to glossary for more information.

Example of Anterior Myocardial Infarction

Acute Anterior MI

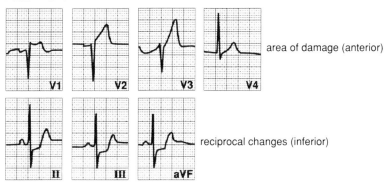

area of damage (anterior)

reciprocal changes (inferior)

Old Anterior MI

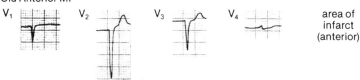

area of
infarct
(anterior)

Q WAVE MYOCARDIAL INFARCTION *(Continued)*

SEPTAL MYOCARDIAL INFARCTION

Cause blockage of the left main or LAD artery
ECG Changes seen in leads V_1 and V_2
- Acute changes are ST elevation.
- Evolving changes are small or no R wave in these leads.

KEY POINTS
- Often occurs with anterior MI (both areas are supplied by the LAD artery in most people).
- Observe for sudden onset of CHF; could possibly be due to septal rupture.

Example of Septal Myocardial Infarction

Acute Septal MI

V₁  V₂   area of
damage
(septal)

I  V₅ V₆ reciprocal
changes
(lateral)

Old Septal MI

V₁  V₂ area of
infarct
(septal)

Q WAVE MYOCARDIAL INFARCTION *(Continued)*

INFERIOR MYOCARDIAL INFARCTION

Cause blockage of the right coronary artery (RCA)
ECG Changes seen in leads II, III, and aVF

Possible Complications after MI dysrhythmias* (specifically PVCs, V-tach, V-fib, or all of these)
pericarditis
CHF
cardiogenic shock
death (usually due to pump failure or myocardial rupture)
ventricular aneurysm

KEY POINTS
- Bradycardias are common with inferior MI because of edema around or ischemia of the upper conduction system (SA node to AV node).
- Because the RCA also supplies blood to the AV node and right ventricle, they too can be affected by diminished blood flow.
- Treatment of an inferior MI depends on the location of the lesion in the RCA; signs of a proximal lesion are:
  – involvement of posterior or lateral wall or both (seen on the ECG as "reciprocal changes")

– development of AV block
– right ventricular infarction (see p. 165)
- Second- or third-degree AV block is often a temporary rhythm lasting 72 to 96 hours; always notify the physician and continue to monitor for dysrhythmias and hemodynamic instability (decreased level of consciousness, skin pale and diaphoretic, anxiety). The slowed ventricular rate and the loss of atrial kick,* rather than AV block, are most threatening to the patient.

---

*Refer to glossary for more information.

Continued on following page

Q WAVE MYOCARDIAL INFARCTION *(Continued)*

Example of Inferior Myocardial Infarction

Acute Inferior MI   II 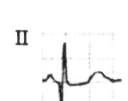   III 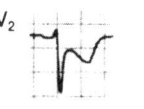   aVF 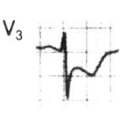   area of damage (inferior)

       V₂ 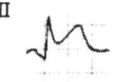   V₃ 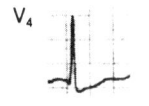   V₄ 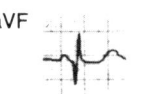   reciprocal changes (anterior)

Old Inferior MI   II 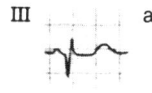   III   aVF   area of infarct (inferior)

RIGHT VENTRICULAR INFARCTION

Clinically, symptoms of a right ventricular (RV) infarct can be classified as "failure without rales" (i.e., signs of CHF but with clear lungs). In this situation the problem is not left ventricular (LV) failure with fluid backing up into the lungs but failure of the RV to pump enough blood to the left side of the heart.

An RV infarct greatly complicates the clinical course of an inferior wall MI, because treatment of one type of failure (e.g., diuretics for peripheral fluid overload from RV compromise) usually worsens the other type of failure (e.g., LV compromise resulting in the need for increased preload, which is treated with fluids).

To check for RV infarct by ECG, obtain a V_4R rhythm strip; ST elevation greater than 1 mm is positive for an RV infarct. The changes disappear in about 8 hours, so obtain the strip on admission. A V_4R strip should be run on *every* patient with suspected inferior wall MI.

Continued on following page

Q WAVE MYOCARDIAL INFARCTION *(Continued)*

Example of Inferior Myocardial Infarction with Right Ventricular Infarction

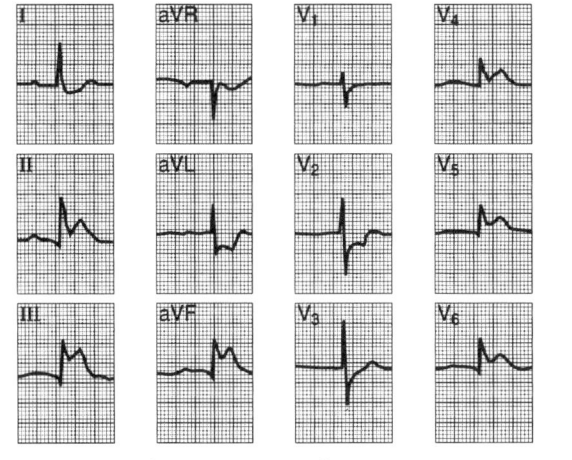

Initial ECG tracing on 6/24 at 6:10 PM.

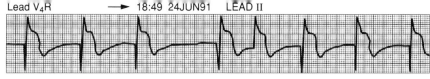

Lead V$_4$R ⟶ 18:49 24JUN91 LEAD II

V$_4$R rhythm strip on 6/24 at 6:49 PM.

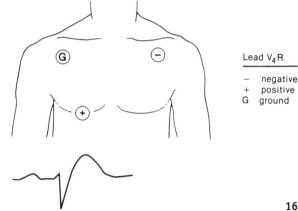

Lead V$_4$R

− negative
+ positive
G ground

V$_4$R with proximal RCA lesion.

167

Q WAVE MYOCARDIAL INFARCTION *(Continued)*

LATERAL MYOCARDIAL INFARCTION

Cause blockage of the diagonal branch of the LAD artery or the circumflex artery in a heart with a dominant RCA

ECG Changes seen in leads I, aVL, V_5, and V_6

KEY POINT Oftentimes lateral MI is associated with anterior MI (both areas are usually supplied by the left coronary artery).

Example of Lateral Myocardial Infarction

Acute Lateral MI

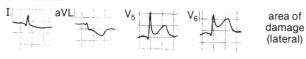

area of
damage
(lateral)

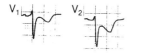

reciprocal
changes
(septal)

Old Lateral MI

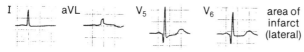

area of
infarct
(lateral)

Q WAVE MYOCARDIAL INFARCTION *(Continued)*

POSTERIOR MYOCARDIAL INFARCTION

Cause blockage of the circumflex artery (branch of the left coronary artery) or posterior
descending branch of a dominant RCA

ECG Changes specific changes seen in leads V_1 and V_2
- tall R wave
- ST depression
- T wave inversion

KEY POINTS
- In the setting of acute inferior MI, these changes may be misinterpreted as reciprocal changes (see Inferior Myocardial Infarction [p. 162] and Right Ventricular Infarction [p. 165]).
- True posterior MIs are rare and are usually uncomplicated.

Acute Posterior MI

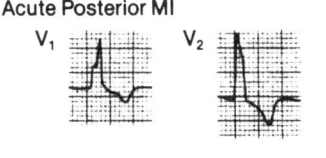

V_1 V_2 area of
damage
(posterior)

NON-Q-WAVE MYOCARDIAL INFARCTION

A non-Q-wave MI usually results either from a spontaneously recanalized artery or from an incomplete occlusion by a thrombus long enough to cause necrosis; it does not affect the entire thickness of the ventricular wall. Changes seen with a non-Q-wave injury or MI affect the same leads as does a Q wave (full-wall thickness) MI; that is, an inferior non-Q-wave MI would be reflected in leads II, III, and aVF.

The acute changes include ST depression and T wave inversion (in affected leads), but no Q waves develop. When first discovered, non-Q-wave MIs were thought to be "small" or inconsequential MIs. It is now believed that the damage is a sign of moderate-to-severe coronary artery disease and can be a heralding sign of a much worse MI.

Example of Non-Q-Wave Myocardial Infarction

Acute non-Q-wave MI

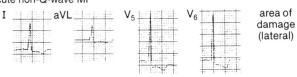

area of
damage
(lateral)

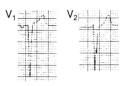

reciprocal
changes
(septal)

CRITICAL LAD STENOSIS (WELLENS SYNDROME)

Definition   characteristic ECG pattern indicating a critical stenosis high (proximal) in the LAD
artery

Patient Presentation   • history of unstable angina
   • changes are seen in pain-free period; patient has not infarcted yet
     (little or no cardiac enzyme elevation)
   • no Q wave
     little or no ST elevation   } in V_2 and V_3
     deeply inverted symmetrical T wave
   • usually ST elevation will be present during pain

KEY POINT   Recognition of these ECG changes signifies a need for an emergency cardiac
catheterization!

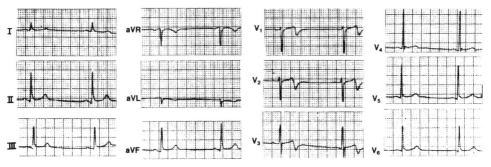

From Wellens HJJ and Conover MB: *The ECG in Emergency Decision Making*. Philadelphia: WB Saunders, 1992.

Continued on following page

CRITICAL LAD STENOSIS (WELLENS SYNDROME) *(Continued)*

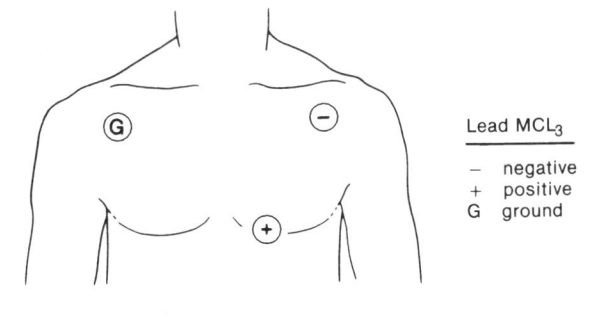

Lead MCL₃

- negative
+ positive
G ground

KEY POINT Because of the importance of recognizing critical LAD stenosis, patients admitted with chest pain should be monitored in lead MCL_3, observing for the ST and T wave changes. Any ECG changes must be verified with a 12-lead ECG.

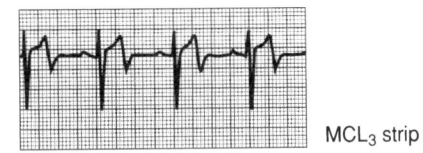

MCL₃ strip taken July 31 of same man as below.

MCL_3 strip

Example of Critical LAD Stenosis (Wellens Syndrome)

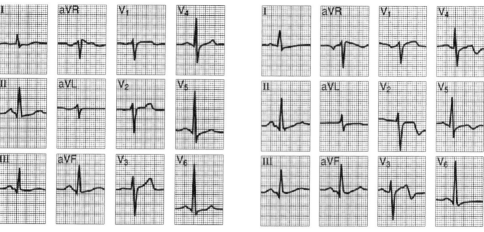

A 65-year-old man admitted with probable non-Q-wave MI on 7/30 at 8:16 AM.

Same patient on 7/31 at 8:14 AM (taken after changes noted on MCL₃ strip [see above]).

◼ Bundle Branch Block (BBB)

Impulses normally are initiated in the SA node, travel to the AV node, and then reach the bundle of His and the right and left bundle branches. The left bundle branch further divides into two fascicles (or branches)—the anterior and the posterior. Blockage of the conduction pathway results in either right bundle branch block (RBBB) or left bundle branch block (LBBB). If only one fascicle of the left bundle branch is affected, it is called a hemiblock,* or a fascicular block (i.e., left anterior hemiblock or left anterior fascicular block). Sometimes, a left anterior hemiblock will occur in conjunction with RBBB, rather than by itself (this is called a bifascicular block).

Possible Causes degenerative disease of the conduction system (e.g., caused by ischemic heart
disease, ventricular hypertrophy,* cardiomyopathy)
acute anterior MI (LBBB or RBBB)
acute inferior MI (RBBB)
cardiac surgery
acute pulmonary embolus (RBBB)

---

*Refer to glossary for more information.

Treatment Treatment of the patient with BBB depends on the type of block and whether it is chronic or acute. A patient with BBB is treated with a pacemaker when the cardiac output is compromised.

- With chronic LBBB or RBBB alone, permanent pacing is not indicated because the cardiac output is not affected by delayed depolarization.*
- When a BBB occurs in an MI setting (especially RBBB with left anterior hemiblock), a temporary pacemaker may be considered, although the physician may wait to see if AV block (Mobitz II or complete) also develops.
- If the patient with LBBB or RBBB does develop Mobitz II or complete AV block, a permanent pacemaker is indicated because the patient's cardiac output is decreased with the slow heart rate associated with the AV block.

---

*Refer to glossary for more information.

Continued on following page

Example of RBBB

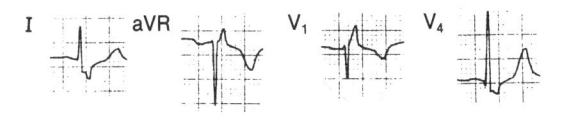

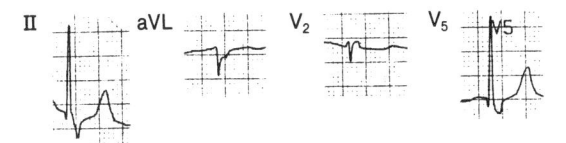

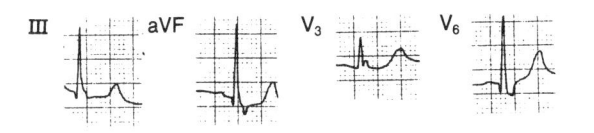

ECG Criteria
- QRS > 0.12 s
- QRS complex in V_1 has rSR′ configuration
- S wave in V_5 and V_6 is broad and slurred

Example of LBBB

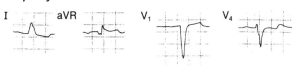

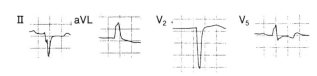

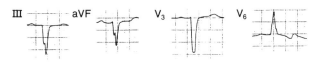

ECG Criteria
- QRS > 0.12 s
- small R wave and deep prolonged S wave in V_1 or V_2 or in both
- slow progression of R wave until V_5 and V_6, at which point it is notched

KEY POINT Because of the ECG changes caused by the LBBB, diagnosis of acute MI by ECG is often difficult, if not impossible.

◼ Differentiating Ectopy and Aberrancy

An aberrant beat originates supraventricularly but is conducted abnormally through the ventricles; the QRS complex has a bundle branch configuration.

An ectopic beat originates in the ventricles; the QRS complex is wide and bizarre looking.

Because both aberrant and ectopic beats are wide, it is sometimes difficult to determine the origin of a tachycardia when it develops. A systematic approach *must* be used!

Do *not* use (because they are not consistently helpful):
- rate of tachycardia
- regularity of tachycardia
- hemodynamic stability or instability
- age of patient

Do use:
- QRS configuration and width (using at least V_1, and sometimes V_2 and V_6)
- presence of precordial concordance (all of the precordial leads are negative or positive)
  – positive concordance suggests V-tach
  – negative concordance is diagnostic of V-tach
- axis (axis in "no man's land" [i.e., negative QRS in both leads I and II] strongly indicates V-tach)
- presence of AV dissociation (present in 50% of V-tach)

When V_1 is predominantly *positive*:

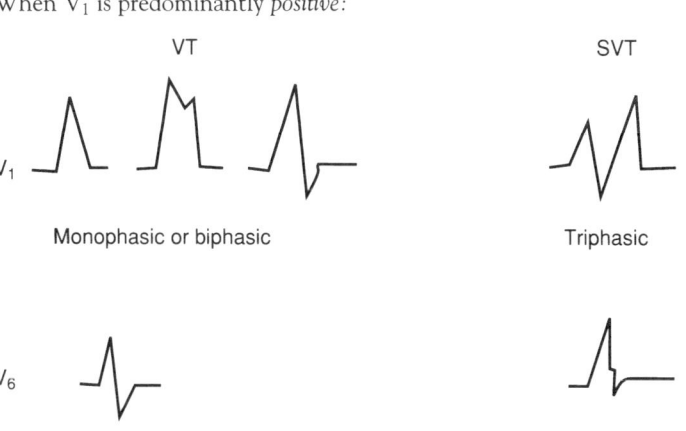

When V₁ is predominantly *negative*:

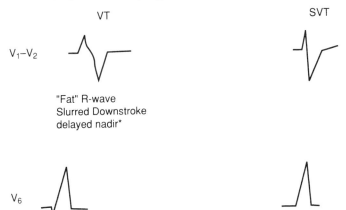

VT

V₁–V₂

"Fat" R-wave
Slurred Downstroke
delayed nadir*

V₆

SVT

*The nadir is the point of the S wave; in ectopic beats, from the onset of the QRS complex to the nadir is >0.06 second.

◣ Digitalis Toxicity

ANTIARRHYTHMIC EFFECTS OF DIGITALIS

Normal slows conduction in the conduction system
        lengthens refractory period* in conduction system

Toxic increases automaticity* ⎫
        increases sympathetic stimulation to heart ⎬ increased tendency for ectopy*
        disturbs AV conduction (can result in AV blocks) ⎭

FACTORS INFLUENCING OCCURRENCE OF TOXICITY

1. therapeutic and toxic doses are close, even more so with advanced cardiac disease
2. electrolyte imbalances (especially hypokalemia)
3. drug interactions (many; some examples are quinidine, amiodarone, calcium channel blockers, sympathetic system stimulants [beta agonists like albuterol], benzodiazepines, diuretics)
4. renal disease (70% of digoxin is excreted renally)
5. hypothyroidism

---

*Refer to glossary for more information.

CLINICAL SIGNS AND SYMPTOMS

GI anorexia, nausea/vomiting

Neurologic headache, fatigue, malaise, confusion, depression

Visual yellow or green halos, blurred vision, colors "just don't look right" (ask patient about newspaper or magazine print and colors on TV)

Cardiac (may have two or more dysrhythmias concurrently)
1. first ECG changes are often prolonged PR interval and ST depression
2. dysrhythmia "alerts" (investigate any *new* rhythm)
   - bradycardia when heart rate had been normal or fast
   - tachycardia when heart rate had been normal
   - regular rhythm in patient known to have an irregular rhythm (e.g., A-fib)
   - regular irregularity
3. dysrhythmias arising from any part of the heart (myocardial cells or conduction system); samples of common ones follow

Continued on following page

Treatment   1. early recognition of rhythms due to toxicity
2. stop digitalis
3. monitor and correct any electrolyte disturbance
4. may treat dysrhythmias with lidocaine* or phenytoin
5. potentially life-threatening toxicity may be treated with digoxin immune fab (Digibind)
6. the relationship of serum digoxin levels to signs and symptoms of intoxication vary widely from patient to patient

---

*For more information on drug therapy, refer to drug section.

JUNCTIONAL TACHYCARDIA (NONPAROXYSMAL)

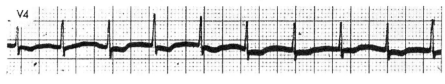

From Braunwald E (ed): *Heart Disease: A Textbook of Cardiovascular Medicine* (2nd ed.). Philadelphia: WB Saunders, 1984, p. 240.

P Waves absent *or* inverted (II) or upright (MCL_1)
Rhythm ventricular, usually regular
Rate 70 to 140 bpm (ventricular)
PR AV dissociation usually present because of digitalis-induced AV block
QRS 0.04 to 0.10 s

KEY POINTS There are several ways in which junctional tachycardia may present:
- junctional rhythm with rate of 70 to 140 bpm
- A-fib with regular ventricular rhythm (digitalis-induced total AV block)
- atrial flutter with AV dissociation due to digitalis-induced AV block—recognize by an inconsistent relationship between flutter waves and the QRS complex

ATRIAL TACHYCARDIA WITH BLOCK

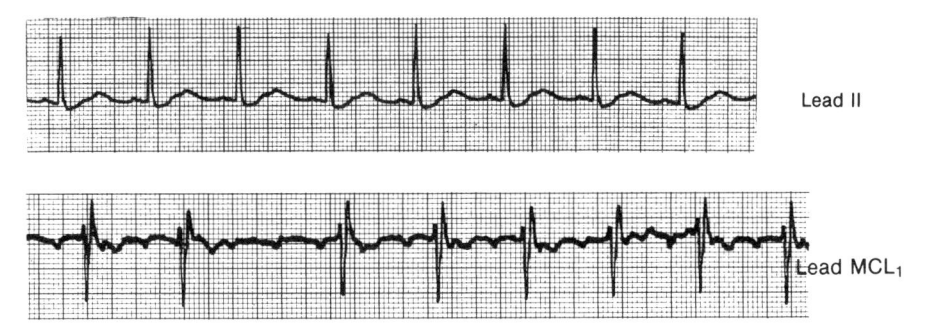

P Waves   similar, usually 2:1 ratio with QRS
             upright in lead II (best lead to use for this rhythm)
Rhythm   atrial, regular or irregular; PP intervals are often ventriculophasic (PP surrounding a
             QRS is shorter than PP without a QRS)
             ventricular, usually regular

Rate atrial, 150 to 250 bpm
ventricular, depends on conduction ratio*
PR usually 0.12 to 0.20 s; constant for conducted P waves
QRS 0.04 to 0.10 s
QT 0.32 to 0.44 s

KEY POINTS
- If this rhythm is not recognized as due to digitalis toxicity, the mortality is 100%.
- When the digitalis is stopped, the ventricular rate may temporarily increase, since conduction through the AV node is improved. This is a positive sign; it is not necessary to notify the physician unless the patient becomes hemodynamically unstable!

---

*Refer to glossary for more information.

■ Glossary

aberrant ventricular conduction Conduction of an impulse *not* by the normal ventricular conduction system (i.e., AV node, bundle of His, bundle branches, and Purkinje fibers) but either through the cardiac muscle itself or through accessory (extra) conduction pathways. The impulse originates supraventricularly, but the QRS will be wide (>0.12 second). Examples of aberrant (or abnormal) ventricular conduction include

- A premature beat (e.g., premature atrial contraction) early enough that not all of the ventricular conduction system has had time to repolarize and thus cannot accept the impulse, so it is conducted aberrantly.
- Conduction through an accessory pathway that bypasses the AV node and thus sends impulses to ventricles faster than is normal (as seen in Wolff-Parkinson-White syndrome). (See also Preexcitation Syndrome in this glossary.)
- A bundle branch block with impulses reaching the affected ventricle by spreading through the muscle tissue.

accelerated escape rhythm Occurs when a lower pacemaker initiates impulses at a rate faster than its inherent rate. Examples include

- A junctional rhythm with rate >60 bpm (remember the inherent junctional rate is 40 to 60 bpm, so a rate >60 bpm is "accelerated").
- A ventricular rhythm with a rate of 80 bpm (see section on Accelerated Idioventricular Rhythm [p. 76]).

atrial kick Contraction of the atria propels blood into the ventricles; that volume of blood is approximately 25% of the amount ejected from the heart with each beat. "Atrial kick" is lost either when atrial contraction does not occur (i.e., with A-fib) or when it is not coordinated with ventricular contraction (i.e., with junctional rhythm or AV dissociation). In patients with borderline cardiac function the loss of 25% of cardiac output can seriously impair hemodynamic stability.

automaticity Spontaneous initiation of impulses by myocardial cells without their waiting for a trigger from the conduction system.

AV dissociation The atria and ventricles are being paced independently (see section on AV Dissociation [p. 93]).

bigeminy Pairs of beats, most often a sinus beat with an early impulse. It usually refers to a PVC every other beat, but it can also be PACs or PJCs. When the bigeminy involves impulses other than PVCs, it is usually stated (i.e., atrial bigeminy).

bradydysrhythmia Rhythm with a ventricular rate <60 bpm. It includes sinus bradycardia as well as abnormal rhythms.

Continued on following page

cardioversion The use of synchronized shock to convert life-threatening tachycardias. When the defibrillator is properly synchronized, the current will be delivered on the R wave, which decreases the chance of accidentally hitting the T wave and converting the rhythm to V-fib. According to AHA guidelines for adults, the initial cardioversion for V-tach is at 100 J; subsequent shocks are at increasing joules (i.e., 200, 300, and up to 360 J). When cardioversion is performed for a PSVT, AHA guidelines suggest starting at 50 J; subsequent shocks are at 100, 200, 300, and 360 J.

carotid sinus massage Massage over the carotid artery that stimulates the vagus nerve and thus creates a vagal response. It is used to slow down or convert tachydysrhythmias to a more normal rhythm. CSM should be done only on a *monitored* patient and *only* by an experienced person.

conpensatory pause Commonly occurs with PVCs because the premature beat does not interfere with the SA node's timing. On an ECG strip, measure the distance between the normal complex before and after the PVC; this distance should be the same as between any three normal complexes.

conduction ratio Denotes more than one atrial contraction for each ventricular contraction. Examples follow:

- Atrial flutter with three flutter waves to each QRS is called "atrial flutter with 3:1 conduction."
- Second-degree AV block with every other P wave conducted is called "second-degree AV block with 2:1 conduction."

A conduction ratio may be constant (as in examples) or altering, as in atrial flutter with 3:1 and 4:1 conduction.

defibrillation Unsynchronized shock to convert a life-threatening dysrhythmia to a more normal rhythm; it is used to treat V-fib and V-tach without a pulse. The AHA guidelines are

- Initial shock at 200 J; second shock at 200 to 300 J. } adult
- Subsequent shocks at up to 360 J.
- Children are defibrillated at 2 J/kg body weight.

depolarization The spread of the electrical impulse through the heart muscle before contraction; atrial depolarization is represented by the P wave, and the ventricular depolarization, by the QRS complex.

Continued on following page

diastolic filling time Systole is contraction of the ventricles; diastole is relaxation of the ventricles, when they fill with blood. As the heart rate increases, diastole shortens, leaving less time for the ventricles to fill. When the ventricles do not fill completely, less blood is ejected into the body and the cardiac output drops. This can be a serious complication in patients with borderline cardiac function who need all their potential cardiac output. Examples of this include
  • Patient develops rapid A-fib and becomes dizzy and hypotensive.
  • Patient feels faint, and monitor shows patient having runs of paroxysmal atrial tachycardia.

dysrhythmia Any ECG rhythm other than sinus rhythm.

ectopic beat An extra or early beat originating in any tissue other than the SA node. "Ectopy" is the presence of "ectopic beats"; for example, PVCs can also be called ventricular ectopy.

hemiblock Blockage of one of the fascicles (branches) of the left bundle branch.
  • Blockage of the anterior fascicle results in left anterior hemiblock or left anterior fascicular block.
  • Blockage of the posterior fascicle results in left posterior hemiblock or left posterior fascicular block.

There are specific ECG and axis changes associated with fascicular blocks. Refer to references for additional resources.

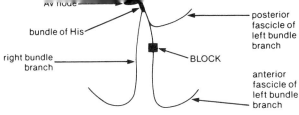

Anterior hemiblock.

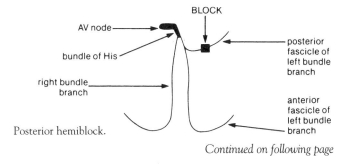

Posterior hemiblock.

Continued on following page

hypertrophy (chamber) Enlargement of the heart (both in muscle mass and chamber size). Possible causes include
- Chronic CHF; the heart increases in size to compensate for poor contractility of ventricles.
- Valvular disease, for example, aortic stenosis; the heart increases in size to try to increase blood flow through narrowed valve.

multiform Impulses originating from more than one focus; the complexes will look different.

preexcitation syndrome A condition in which there is an accessory (extra) pathway that bypasses all or part of the AV node or bundle of His, thus allowing atrial impulses to depolarize ventricular muscle earlier than if they were traveling via the normal conduction system. Dysrhythmias associated with preexcitation syndromes include tachycardias, rapid A-fib, rapid atrial flutter, V-fib, and occasionally V-tach. An example of preexcitation syndrome is Wolff-Parkinson-White syndrome. In this case the Kent bundle allows atrial impulses to bypass the AV node and thus reach the ventricles quickly (see figure below).

radiofrequency ablation Radiofrequency energy is delivered to a part of the conduction system by a catheter to cause scarring; used to treat SVT, A-fib, atrial flutter, and V-tach.

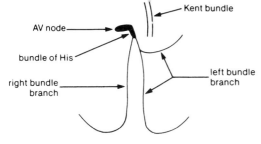

Preexcitation syndrome.

Continued on following page

199

reentry phenomenon Usually occurs at the level of the Purkinje fibers or junctional tissue. Reentry can occur when there is a bifurcation in the conduction pathway and a unidirectional (one-way) block in one limb of the bifurcation. When the impulse reaches the bifurcation, it can only go down the limb that is not blocked (A in illustration below). After depolarizing the tissue distal to the bifurcation, the impulse can return through the blocked limb (because the block is only in one direction) and reenter the tissue that was previously inexcitable but that can now be depolarized (B in illustration). The reentry impulse can then depolarize tissue before an impulse has time to come from the SA node (C in illustration). If this reentry phenomenon is maintained, a tachycardia develops. Reentry is thought to be a possible cause of PVCs, V-tach, and V-fib, as well as supraventricular tachydysrhythmias.

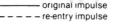
———— original impulse
— — — re-entry impulse

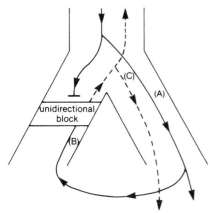

unidirectional
block

(C)

(A)

(B)

Reentry phenomenon.

refractory period The time during which the tissue (e.g., atrial cells, conduction system, ventricular cells) cannot accept another impulse.

reperfusion The return of blood flow to an area of myocardium supplied by the previously occluded artery. Common dysrhythmias associated with reperfusion include accelerated idioventricular rhythm, bradycardia, PVCs, and occasionally V-tach.

repolarization The "resting state" of myocardial cells when they prepare themselves for another depolarization. Ventricular repolarization is represented on the ECG by the T wave; atrial repolarization occurs but is obscured on the ECG by the QRS complex.

standardized 12-lead ECG An ECG in which a 1 mV electrical impulse causes a positive deflection of 10 mm on the ECG paper (ten small squares), and the paper speed is 25 mm/s. This is the normal 12-lead ECG.

tachydysrhythmia An abnormal rhythm with a ventricular rate >100 bpm.

thrombolytic therapy Medications given to "dissolve" clots, usually in the coronary arteries. Common thrombolytic agents include streptokinase, alteplase (t-PA), and reteplase.

uniform Impulses originating from one focus; the complexes look alike.

American Heart Association: *Textbook for Advanced Cardiac Life Support*. Dallas: American Heart Association, 1990.

Bennett JC and Plum F (eds): *Cecil Textbook of Medicine*, 20th ed. Philadelphia: WB Saunders, 1996.

Conover M: Wellens syndrome: Identification of critical proximal left anterior descending stenosis. *Critical Care Nurse* 10:30–36, 1990.

Conover M: *Understanding Electrocardiography*, 7th ed. St. Louis: CV Mosby, 1996.

Hill NE and Goodman JS: Importance of accurate placement of precordial leads in the 12-lead electrocardiogram. *Heart and Lung* 16(5):561–566, 1987.

Josephson ME and Wellens IIJJ: Differential diagnosis of supraventricular tachycardia. *Cardiology Clinics* 8:411–442, 1990.

Kinney MR, Packa D, Andreoli K, and Zipes D: *Comprehensive Cardiac Care*, 8th ed. St. Louis: CV Mosby, 1996.

Lundberg GD: Guidelines for cardiopulmonary resuscitation and emergency cardiac care. *Journal of American Medical Association* 268(16):2199–2241, 1992.

Marriott HJL: *Practical Electrocardiography*, 8th ed. Baltimore: Williams & Wilkins, 1988.

Olin BR (ed): *Drug Facts and Comparisons*. St. Louis: Wolters Kluwer, 1997.

Phillips RE and Feeney MK: *The Cardiac Rhythms: A Systematic Approach to Interpretation*, 3rd ed. Philadelphia: WB Saunders, 1990.

Wellens HJJ and Conover MB: *The ECG in Emergency Decision Making*. Philadelphia: WB Saunders, 1992.

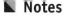 **Notes**

Notes

Aberrant beat, 182–183
Aberrant ventricular conduction, 192
Accelerated escape rhythm, 192
Accelerated idioventricular rhythm, 76–77
Accelerated junctional rhythm, 54–56
ACLS algorithms, 120–135
    for asystole, 130
    for bradycardia, 132–133
    for pulseless electrical activity, 128–129
    for pulseless ventricular tachycardia,
        122–123
    for supraventricular tachycardia, 134–135
    for ventricular fibrillation, 122–123
    for wide-QRS tachycardia, 124–127
Adenosine (Adenocard), 98
Adrenalin (epinephrine), 108–109
Amrinone (Inocor), 99
Asystole, 72–73
Atrial fibrillation, 44–46
Atrial flutter, 42–43

Atrial rate, 9
Atrial tachycardia, with block, 190–191
Atrioventricular block, first-degree, 78–79
    identification of, 92
    second-degree, Mobitz I (Wenckebach),
        80–82
        Mobitz II, 84–86
    third-degree (complete), 88–90
Atrioventricular dissociation, 93, 193
Atrioventricular node, rate of, 10
Atrium, abnormalities of, 144–147
Atropine, 100
Automaticity, 193
Axis, for 12-lead electrocardiogram, 140–141

Betapace (dl-sotalol), 105
Bigeminy, 193
Bradycardia, 16
    ACLS algorithm for, 132–133
Bradycardia-tachycardia syndrome, 34

Bretylium (Bretylol), 101
Bundle branch block, 178–181

Calan (verapamil), 119
Calcium chloride, 102
Cardiac arrest, ACLS algorithms for, 120–135
Cardioversion, 126–127, 194
Cardizem Lyo-Ject (diltiazem), 104
Carotid sinus massage, 194
Catecholamines, 95, 106, 107, 108–109, 111
Compensatory pause, 194
Conduction ratio, 195
Conduction system, 2
    delays in, 16
    normal activity of, 3
Corvert (ibutilide fumarate), 110
Critical LAD stenosis (Wellens syndrome),
        174–177

Defibrillation, 195
Depolarization, 195

Diastolic filling time, 196
Digitalis toxicity, 186–191
Digoxin (Lanoxin), 103
Diltiazem (Cardizem Lyo-Ject), 104
Dobutamine (Dobutrex), 106
Dopamine (Intropin), 107
Drugs, cardiac, 94–119. See also specific
        drugs.
    mechanism of action of, 96–97
Dysrhythmia, 196
    risk factors for, 16

Ectopic beats, 16, 182–183, 196
Electrocardiogram, 136–143, 202
    axis determination for, 140–141
    electrodes for, 12–15, 137–139
    in accelerated idioventricular rhythm, 76–77
    in accelerated junctional rhythm, 54–56
    in anterior myocardial infarction, 158–159
    in asystole, 72–73
    in atrial fibrillation, 44–46

Electrocardiogram *(Continued)*
   in atrial flutter, 42–43
   in bundle branch block, 178–181
   in critical LAD stenosis (Wellens
      syndrome), 174–177
   in first-degree atrioventricular block,
      78–79
   in idioventricular rhythm, 74–75
   in inferior myocardial infarction, 162–164
   in junctional rhythm, 50–52
   in lateral myocardial infarction, 168–169
   in left atrial abnormality, 146–147
   in left ventricular hypertrophy, 152–153
   in Mobitz I (Wenckebach) second-degree
      atrioventricular block, 80–82
   in Mobitz II second-degree atrioventricular
      block, 84–86
   in multifocal atrial tachycardia, 40–41
   in non-Q-wave myocardial infarction,
      172–173

Electrocardiogram *(Continued)*
   in normal sinus rhythm, 20–22
   in posterior myocardial infarction, 170
   in premature atrial contraction, 36–37
   in premature junctional contraction, 48–49
   in premature ventricular contraction, 60–63
   in Q wave myocardial infarction, 154–170
   in right atrial abnormality, 144–145
   in right ventricular hypertrophy, 150–151
   in right ventricular infarction, 165–167
   in septal myocardial infarction, 160–161
   in sick sinus syndrome, 34
   in sinus arrest, 32–33
   in sinus bradycardia, 24–25
   in sinus dysrhythmia, 28–29
   in sinus exit block, 30–31
   in sinus tachycardia, 26–27
   in supraventricular tachycardia, 58–59
   in third-degree (complete) atrioventricular
      block, 88–90

Electrocardiogram (*Continued*)
  in torsades de pointes, 68–69
  in ventricular fibrillation, 70–71
  in ventricular hypertrophy, 148–153
  in ventricular tachycardia, 64–67
  in wandering atrial pacemaker, 38–39
  interpretation of, 18
  normal, 142–143
Electrodes, for electrocardiogram, 12–15,
    137–139
Epinephrine (Adrenalin), 95, 108–109
Escape rhythm, accelerated, 192

Hemiblock, 196–197
Hypertrophy, 198

Ibutilide fumarate (Corvert), 110
Idioventricular rhythm, 74–75
  accelerated, 76–77
Inderal (propranolol), 116
Inocor (amrinone), 99

Intervals, 6–7
Intropin (dopamine), 107
Isoproterenol (Isuprel), 111
Isoptin (verapamil), 119

Junctional rhythm, 50–52
  accelerated, 54–56
Junctional tachycardia, nonparoxysmal, 189

LAD stenosis (Wellens syndrome), 174–177
Lanoxin (digoxin), 103
Leads, 12–13
  limb, 137
  precordial, 138–139
  reversal of, 14–15
Lead II, 12, 14
Lead MCL_1, 13, 15
Left bundle branch block, 178–181
Left ventricular hypertrophy, 152–153
Lidocaine, 112
Limb leads, 137

Magnesium sulfate, 113
MCL_1 lead, 13, 15
Morphine, 114
Multifocal atrial tachycardia, 40–41
Multiform impulses, 198
Myocardial infarction, anterior, 158–159
   inferior, 162–164
   lateral, 168–169
   non-Q-wave, 172–173
   posterior, 170
   Q wave, 154–170
   right ventricular, 165–167
   septal, 160–161

Nonparoxysmal junctional tachycardia, 189
Normal sinus rhythm, 20–22

P mitrale, 146–147
P pulmonale, 144–145
P wave, 4
   in ECG rhythm strip interpretation, 18

Pacemakers, natural, 10
PR interval, 5
   in ECG rhythm strip interpretation, 18
   measurement of, 6
   normal, 7
Precordial leads, 138–139
Preexcitation syndrome, 198, 199
Premature atrial contraction, 36–37
Premature junctional contraction, 48–49
Premature ventricular contraction, 60–63
Procainamide (Pronestyl, Procan SR), 115
Propranolol (Inderal), 116
Pulseless electrical activity, ACLS algorithm
   for, 128–129

QRS complex, 4
   axis of, 140–141
   in wide-QRS tachycardia, 184–185
   normal, 7
QRS interval, 5
   in ECG rhythm strip interpretation, 18

QT interval, 5, 7
  in ECG rhythm strip interpretation, 18
  normal, 7
Quinidine, 117

R wave, in rate calculation, 8
Radiofrequency ablation, 198
Rates, calculation of, 8–9
Reentry phenomenon, 200–201
Refractory period, 202
Reperfusion, 202
Repolarization, 202
Right bundle branch block, 178–181
Right ventricular hypertrophy, 150–151

Sick sinus syndrome, 34
Sinoatrial block, second-degree, 30–31
Sinoatrial node, rate of, 10
Sinus arrest, 32–33
Sinus bradycardia, 21, 24–25

Sinus dysrhythmia, 28–29
Sinus exit block, 30–31
Sinus rhythm, normal, 20–22
Sinus tachycardia, 21, 26–27
Sodium bicarbonate, 118
dl-Sotalol (Betapace), 105
Supraventricular tachycardia, 58–59
  ACLS algorithm for, 134–135

T wave, 4
Tachycardia, 16
  atrial, multifocal, 40–41
    with block, 190–191
  junctional, nonparoxysmal, 189
  sinus, 21, 26–27
  supraventricular, 58–59, 134–135
  ventricular, 64–67, 122–127
    pulseless, 122–123
  wide-QRS, 124–127, 184–185
Tachydysrhythmia, 202

Thrombolytic therapy, 202
Torsades de pointes, 68–69

Uniform impulses, 202

Ventricular fibrillation, 70–71
   ACLS algorithm for, 122–123
Ventricular hypertrophy, 148–153
   pathogenesis of, 148–149
Ventricular rate, 8–9, 10
Ventricular tachycardia, 64–67
   ACLS algorithm for, 122–127

Ventricular tachycardia *(Continued)*
   cardioversion for, 126–127
   pulseless, ACLS algorithm for, 122–123
Verapamil (Calan, Isoptin), 119

Wandering atrial pacemaker, 38–39
Waveforms, 4
Wellens syndrome (critical LAD stenosis),
   174–177
Wide-QRS tachycardia, 124–127
   QRS configurations in, 184–185